Autism:

"A Family Lives Beyond the Label"

The Lindsey Moreland Story

By Lindsey Moreland, Lauri Moreland,

Todd Moreland, Brittany Moreland,

And Ida Feyereisen

Writing support and direction

From Linda Wagner

Autism:

"A Family Lives Beyond the Label"
The Lindsey Moreland Story
Copyright © 2017

Cover Art by Lindsey Moreland

ISBN: 978-0-9993488-0-2

Second Printing: May, 2018- 1,000 copies

Please visit the Moreland Family website at

www.autismlm.com

Printed in the USA by

Morris Publishing®

3212 E. Hwy. 30 ● Kearney, NE 68847

800-650-7888 ● www.morrispublishing.com

Foreword

This is my daughter Lindsey Moreland's story, written by Lindsey, her grandmother Ida, her dad Todd, her sister Brittany, and me. Autism: A Family Living Beyond the Label is purposely written in short chapters in no particular order to reflect the often unpredictable life many children with autism experience. We hope you won't find this confusing. Through our memories and experiences, you may laugh, cry, and feel emotionally connected, but most of all we hope you are encouraged. Our hope had always been to someday publish her story. We had no idea how her life would progress, but we felt we had many things to say that might help other children and adults with autism, their parents, and educators.

Our daughter Brittany was almost 3 years old when her sister was born. There is no doubt she struggled with her sister's behavior from the very beginning. At the age of 10, Brittany had her first grand mal seizure. Epilepsy added many new struggles to her own physical, mental, and emotional health, yet she put her own issues aside so many times to be there for Lindsey. In writing this book, we are not trying to make Lindsey's story more important than Brittany's, but with the increasing number of children being diagnosed with autism every year, it seems important to publish this book now in 2017.

Our family has been fortunate to have many positive influences in our lives, including a large extended family, friends, teachers, mentors, and therapists. I sincerely believe that all of these people have helped Lindsey become the person she is today.

Lauri Moreland

Table of Contents

Chapter One

"What is autism?"

By Lindsey Moreland

"You have autism," my mom said one day as we were sitting at home. I was crying and feeling bad about school and friends. I remember being in seventh grade, and school was just so hard. It was not just the subjects that challenged me. I could handle math, reading, and writing with some help. However, it was socializing that was difficult. Where should I sit at lunch? Who would want to sit by me? Who would be my partner when the teacher tells the class to find a partner? Would I once again be the last one chosen as other students look around searching for their best friend? Why can't the teacher just pick our partners and save me this agony of worrying? Who will I sit by on the bus? Will I walk up and down the aisle asking, "Can I sit by you?" Will their familiar response be, "No. I am saving this for someone," or "We don't have room." These were my daily concerns. These were the thoughts that I cried about, and my mom, dad, and family helped me deal with day after day and year after year. This is not the beginning of my story. I didn't just wake up in middle school and have autism. Yet, it's my first memory of hearing the word. It is not the end of my story either.

"What is autism?" I wondered. I had absolutely no idea. I just knew that it meant I didn't have friends right now and I didn't know how to make them. In my mind, autism meant having no friends. Autism meant I was odd, different, and basically not normal.

I am Lindsey Moreland. I have autism. Today, is June 11, 2016. I am 22 years old, and today just happens to be my mom's 48th birthday. (You might wonder why I am adding the date. Dates are important to me and you will discover that as you read on.) I have learned a lot about autism and who I am. I am happy to be the person I am today. Autism does not go away, but I have learned how to live with it. This is my story. Everything you will read, whether sad, funny, happy, or concerning, has been approved by me.

Chapter Two

"PDD! Thank goodness she doesn't have autism!"

By Lauri Moreland, Lindsey's mom

It was a cold, December day. Snow covered the ground. I don't remember if I had lunch ready for my two daycare kids and my own two girls. And, I don't remember if the laundry was piled up or not. I do remember that day after day I waited to hear from the Child Health Specialty Clinic in Iowa with regards to an appointment Lindsey had because of her disturbing behaviors and developmental delays. It had been four weeks and I had heard nothing. Brittany, our 4 year old daughter, was playing with Al, one of my daycare kids. They were taking turns driving a little red car in the basement. Lindsey, at 18 months old, was playing in the bathtub in the middle of the day. It was a typical day of screaming for Lindsey, and this was all I could offer her in order to calm her down. She had her swimsuit on, and I was relieved to have at most ten minutes free from one of her tantrums. I went to get the mail out of the mail slot right outside the living room door in our 1950's home in Clear Lake, Iowa.

The mail of the day consisted of bills and some junk mail fliers. Amongst it, was a business envelope from North Iowa Early Intervention. I was numb. I had wondered if I would ever hear from them. I expected a phone call, not a letter. Now, here I stood with a letter in my hands that could potentially change our lives forever. I walked to the kitchen and opened it. Skimming over the letter, I searched for the diagnosis. It said that Lindsey possibly had Pervasive Developmental Disorder. The diagnosis was made after one visit with a specialist, but after many months of concern. I said, "Good, it's not autism." I set the letter on the counter and went on with my day just trying to survive. Little did I know at the time, that PDD is autism. I was 27 years old, married to my high school sweetheart Todd, had two beautiful girls, a house, yet I still felt broken. There was something wrong with my little girl Lindsey, but in my mind at least it wasn't autism.

When Todd came home that night, I told him that we got a letter that said Lindsey didn't have autism. He had little to no reaction which didn't surprise me. Todd hadn't seen enough of what I saw each day because he was working a lot. Also, no matter how hard I tried to explain to him what was going on with Lindsey, I felt like he didn't hear me or want to hear me. I didn't look up what PDD was. This was years before I would learn to ask for clarifying questions and become an advocate for Lindsey. A couple of days later when I was going through the mail, I tossed that letter into the garbage.

Chapter Three

"Healthy, what is healthy?"

By Ida Feyereisen, Lindsey's Grandma

Many times I've heard expectant parents say it doesn't matter if they have a boy or girl, as long as he or she is healthy. HEALTHY? Just what do we mean by healthy? We expect crying, eating, wetting, soft and gentle breathing, and a pink complexion. The baby should be examined by the doctor, have good vital signs, and receive a good Apgar score.

Lindsey met all those requirements, therefore she was pronounced healthy. What a special day! It was January 16, 1994 and Lindsey Maddie Moreland was born on her Great Grandmother Mathilda's 89th birthday. Almost three-year-old Brittany now had the little sister she was hoping for, and we had the 7th of what would eventually be our 15 grandchildren.

The thought that a hospital would even consider sending a two-day-old baby home when wind chills were topping seventy degrees below zero was upsetting to me. What if the car stalled? But, of course it didn't, and their family was now all warm and cozy with us in our home. I was enjoying every minute of this short time Lauri, Todd and the girls would be living with us. Lauri had come back to the room she had shared with her sister, Linda, as a child. This was the second time in their six years of marriage that Todd and she would be living with us. The first time they lived with us, Lauri was on bedrest during the final months of her pregnancy with Brittany. She would again be returning, not only as our child, but also as a wife, mother, and a real adult friend.

Lauri was on partial bedrest during the end of her pregnancy with Lindsey. However, their real reason to live with us this time was very different. Their house in Wisconsin had sold fast. Soon their new home would be ready for them in Iowa, where Todd was relocated for work. It was only a two and a half hour drive away, but to us it would be monumental.

I have been asked when I first heard the word autism. It was several months before Lindsey was born. I was watching a television program where they were interviewing families with children that had behavior issues. The parents on the program were talking about their daughter and showed a video clip of her. The girl appeared to be about 10-12 years old and seemed to be afraid of life. The image that stuck in my mind was the girl standing in the corner with her back to the rest of the people in the room. She wouldn't come when she was called, she didn't respond at all to her mother's voice, and her mother said that she was nonverbal. Upset about something, she was screaming, her fists were clenched, and her body was stiff. I sensed that she was either in pain or angry at something or someone. Her mother conveyed that this kind of behavior was part of their everyday life. They called it autism.

I had heard that a friend's granddaughter had recently been diagnosed with autism. The only thing I knew about her diagnosis was that she couldn't speak. Now, remembering back to that short 2-3 minute TV clip, I had a snapshot of what the word meant. My heart sunk. "Could this be what Lindsey has?"

The few weeks that Todd and Lauri had hoped to be with us would turn into almost five months. It was during these early weeks of Lindsey's life that I knew something was wrong. Lindsey's body stiffened and her arms flew with every attempt Lauri made to nurse her. She lost weight, became constipated, cried a lot, slept little, and basically did not want to be touched. I cried inside. Lauri cried outside, and I felt helpless. Soon, after more attempts and rejections than I would have been able to endure, formula in a bottle replaced her mother's milk. Even though the doctor assured Lauri and Todd that there was no stomach or intestinal blockage, and therefore no reason for her not to eat, we all became frustrated.

It was soon evident that Lindsey took the bottle best when she wasn't held. Lauri would put her in her car seat next to the sofa. She would lie on the sofa and hold the bottle over the side for Lindsey. It was sad, but the only thing that worked. Most attempts to hold her ended the same. Pure and simple, she didn't like it. Days and nights were all extremely long. Todd was gone to work during the day, and traveled to Iowa most weekends to work on renovating the beautiful, old home they had purchased. They would make the move when Todd's company relocated.

These five months went fast for me, and the entry in my journal on the day they moved out of our home shows the emptiness I felt. This was the first and only time any of our five grown children and their families would be moving this far away. It would not be long before we realized that Lindsey's health would only add to the frustration of the miles between us.

Chapter Four

"PDD is autism."

By Lauri Moreland, Lindsey's mom

As I reflected on the months that led up to receiving the "PDD letter," I read through Lindsey's stacks and stacks of medical records. It was like opening an old wound. It brought me back to the previous months before the "letter."

It was 1995. The president of the United States was Bill Clinton. O.J. Simpson was on trial for murder, and the whole world was tuned into watch. A gallon of regular gas was $1.15 and a dozen eggs was $1.16. A gallon of milk was $2.69. None of these mattered to me, except for maybe one-the gallon of milk. Lindsey would only drink milk. We could hardly get her to eat anything. Yet, she loved milk. I remember driving two blocks to the store every day when Todd got home from work to buy milk. It was my reason at the time to get out of the house for a few minutes. I could have easily purchased two gallons at a time, but I needed a few minutes alone. As the months went by, I soon joined an exercise gym so that I could get out of the house at night even more. This was the only way I could keep my sanity from the daily struggles with Lindsey.

Since moving to Iowa from Wisconsin, I continued to notice that Lindsey was not developing and progressing the way her sister Brittany had as a toddler. Although Lindsey was making typical to advanced gross motor milestones such as sitting up at 6 months, crawling at 8 months, and walking at 9 ½ months, I had a hard time bonding with her. I tried and tried, but the connection between us was not there. I remember holding Brittany in my arms as a baby, and there was this immediate sense of love that seemed to flow both ways. Sadly, I didn't feel that with Lindsey, and I searched for it every day. She wasn't giving back or even showing me an ounce of affection.

A specific incident at 10 months old led me to take Lindsey to the doctor. It was about 1:00, and she had finished her lunch. I told her that it was time for a nap. Immediately, she walked to the brick wall in our family room and started banging her head on it while crying. I tried to sooth her, but it didn't work. She continued to cry, scream, and throw herself all over. After calling the doctor, I made arrangements for the neighbor to watch Brittany. The screaming and crying did not stop during the car ride or at the doctor's office. In the three hours that we were there, the doctor ran several tests. She had blood work done. They also used a catheter to check to see if she had a bladder infection or if anything else would show up in her urine. Nothing showed up, and after three hours, the doctor handed her a sucker. Lindsey stopped crying, and the words the doctor said to me are etched in my mind forever.

He said, "I am sorry. That was just a tantrum. There is nothing medically wrong with her."

This explosive tantrum was just the beginning of many more tantrums and concerns. About six weeks later, Lindsey was admitted into the hospital because she tore the lining in her stomach and was vomiting up blood. The doctors believed it was due to a flu virus. She remained in the hospital for 24 hours under observation. When I thought things couldn't get worse, they did. We brought Lindsey home, and it seemed as though she was a changed child, not for the better. She lost the few words that she once spoke. She no longer said "Mama," "Dada," "duck," and "hot." Todd and I had a conversation about what we noticed, and we both agreed that she was regressing even more.

I felt like my life was unfair. What did I do wrong to deserve a child who screamed all day? Why couldn't I bond with her? Why did she push me away? The other little girl in my daycare who was the same age was talking and loved playing with other kids. Lindsey's way of communicating with me was to take my hand and pull me into a room, expecting me to know exactly what she wanted. If I couldn't figure it out, she would have a huge tantrum that potentially lasted for hours or even a whole day. I physically had to wrap my arms and legs around her as she sat on my lap so that she would not hurt herself. As she flailed her arms and legs, it took all of my strength to hold her down. It seemed that no one could help her or me. My family and friends were miles and hours away. More than any time in my life, I felt like I needed my mom. I would talk to her on the phone each day. Some days I could fight back the tears, but most days I couldn't. I shared with her how terrible my life had become.

As the tantrums continued and we were at a loss as to what to do, I brought Lindsey back to our family doctor. Upon witnessing several more tantrums, our doctor referred us to North Iowa Early Intervention. We scheduled an appointment for December 18, 1995. The doctor who observed her was a medical practitioner, not a psychologist. From that appointment, he suggested Lindsey have a MRI, a blood level and chromosome study done, and a DNA study for Fragile X Syndrome. We waited to hear the results. Again, the test results read "normal." The diagnosis in the letter was: #1-Possible Pervasive Developmental Disorder and #2-Temper Tantrums.

A few days after I had thrown the letter away which in my mind read, "She does not have autism," I got a phone call from a high school classmate named Susan. I hadn't been friends with her in high school. In fact, we hung out in two totally different crowds. I vaguely remember saying "hi" in the hallway. However, our parents were friends. Susan was the last person I expected to hear from. My mom had told me that Susan had a daughter who had been diagnosed with autism. At the time, I was heartless to it because it didn't affect me, and I had my own life that I was trying to live.

It was the middle of the day when I got that call. The daycare kids were watching a movie. Lindsey was turning the light switch on and off continuously, which drove me crazy. I could have told her to stop, but that would have led to a major tantrum. Susan told me that she had been talking to my mom and heard that we were struggling with Lindsey. She asked how I was doing, and then she started asking more questions.

"What doctors have you seen?"

"What have the doctors been telling you?"

"Are you working with any therapists?" "What are they saying?"

After several more questions, I told her that I got a letter in the mail from a doctor that we had seen four weeks ago.

She asked, "What did the letter say?" I told her I really didn't know for sure and that I threw it in the garbage. She asked, "Did it say autism?"

I replied, "No. It wasn't that." I remembered that we hadn't dumped the kitchen garbage in a few days, so I went into the garbage and dug through it. I found the letter.

"I found it," I said, as I continued talking to her on the phone. She asked me to read it to her. I don't recall what the first couple paragraphs said. I do know that at the end of the letter it said, "I feel that Lindsey Moreland has possible Pervasive Developmental Disorder."

On the other end of the phone I heard a groan from Susan. "I hate when doctors do that. Lauri, PDD is autism."

I was determined to get Lindsey the help she needed. In Iowa, a hearing test was done and it came back normal. Therapy for Lindsey was recommended, and a therapist came to the house once a week for one hour. I wished that I had more help because it just wasn't enough. We completed and followed through on an Individualized Family Service Plan. Brittany was able to get ten sessions of therapy to help her adjust with our family situation. Looking back, I wonder why parents weren't offered therapy as well. I didn't think I needed it at the time, but after hearing from my family that I cried all the time, it probably would have been helpful.

In Iowa, we were also told by the therapist that Lindsey needed to get as much help as possible. The cost would be an issue, though. In their words, it would be "astronomical." SSI (Social Security Income) papers were filled out upon their suggestion. The money that Lindsey would receive would help us purchase equipment for therapy such as a trampoline, ball pit, weighted vest, pillows, and more. Because of Todd's job change and decreased income, she qualified for the money. Monthly, I had to make the call to SSI and report what we were spending the money on, specifically for Lindsey. We were grateful to have the money and used a lot of it on copays for her medical bills.

Through all of these appointments and phone calls, my stress was building and Lindsey continued to struggle. Every night I went to bed with either a book about autism or a stack of medical papers that I truly didn't understand. As a result I almost always cried myself to sleep. How would we survive this?

Chapter Five

"If you're going to keep crying about it, STOP reading about it."

By Todd, Lindsey's dad

I have been asked to talk about when I first heard the word autism. We were living in Iowa and quite honestly the last thing on my mind was what the word meant. I had moved my family of four from our brand new house in Wisconsin to Iowa because the company I worked for, transferred to this location. I was running the shipping department. Unfortunately, when we arrived, the company started going downhill fast. Here I was with an older house that we were fixing up, trying to support my family, and trying to find a new job. On top of it all, I would come home and our youngest daughter Lindsey screamed pretty much 24-7, and my wife was unhappy.

When the company went "belly up," I found a new job as a factory worker in a nearby town. I had to work all of the time with my new job. I worked 12 hour days during the week and 10 hour days on Saturdays. It was mandatory. I worked and I slept. Lauri pretty much had to do everything when it came to the care of our two girls. Basically, we were just trying to survive. I didn't want to think about autism or any other problems. Lauri was doing daycare which I knew she didn't even like, and it brought very little income into the home. This added extra pressure for me to work as much as possible. I hoped that by working I could provide some sort of happiness for my family.

The day Lauri told me about her phone call from her high school classmate Susan, I had stopped at the store after work to pick up meat from the meat market. I made sure to look at the sales of the day. I don't remember what I chose but it was probably Iowa Chops which were two inch thick pork chops. I grilled a lot. It felt like a typical day. I was exhausted from my 12 hour shift, looking forward to having supper, and going to bed. After supper when the girls were downstairs playing, Lauri and I sat in the family room. She talked about the letter and said the word autism. I had never heard of it, and it really meant very little to me. I refused to believe my daughter had anything wrong with her.

"No," I said. "There is nothing wrong with Lindsey." I hadn't seen the tantrums Lauri talked about due to working so much. I thought maybe the crying was because she couldn't hear. I knew that when I said her name, she rarely looked to me. Lauri started crying again, and I had no clue how to help her feel better or to make the situation better.

I went to bed. Lauri stayed up to read, and I guessed she was reading about autism. The days were the same. I worked. I ate. I slept, and Lauri cried. She probably tried to talk to me about autism each day, but I wouldn't have remembered what she said. I continued to try to provide for my family. One night, weeks later, we were lying in bed, and Lauri was crying. Each night was like this, and I was getting frustrated. I was getting less and less sleep every night because she was so upset. My days were getting harder and harder. Again, Lauri was reading in bed about autism. She was crying, and she wouldn't stop. I didn't know what to say.

I said, "If you're going to keep crying about it, STOP reading about it."

Chapter Six

"It's a roller coaster with twists and turns."

By Brittany Moreland, Lindsey's Sister

The first thing I remember from my childhood was Christmas Eve when I was 5 years old. It is a vivid, heart wrenching memory that will always stick with me. We were living in Iowa. It was supposed to be the happiest of times, yet it wasn't. I had a mom, a dad, and the little sister that I always dreamed of having. Everyone loves Christmas. I was excited to open a gift from my Great Grandma Feyereisen, the same great grandma who shared Lindsey's birthday. She was also the same great grandma who I would later spend a lot of time with due to Lindsey's autism and therapy.

The present was a Barbie Sea World doll complete with a wet suit and a seal. Overjoyed, I was anxious to see what Lindsey got from Great Grandma. Great Grandma Feyereisen always called Lindsey her "Little Honey Bunches." Lindsey's present was a boy Barbie Sea World doll with a dolphin. The noises from Lindsey's mouth were short, sharp, and gurgled as she slammed the Barbie to the ground. I wondered what she was going to do as she got up and headed towards the brick wall. She began banging her head on the brick wall. Mom was telling her to stop, and I was crying. I was scared.

I said, "What's wrong with Lindsey? I will switch presents if that helps."

Days later, the whole family went to the doctor with Lindsey. While mom was with Lindsey, my dad was playing with me in the waiting room. I remember how much fun I was having that day with my dad, playing with a toy that resembled a roller coaster with twists and turns, loops, and it even went upside down. Years later, you could say that is kind of how our life was back then, living with a sister who has autism.

Lindsey came out of the doctor's office with a sticker and a sucker. The look on my mom's face was confusing. I could feel her frustration.

My mom said, "They don't know what is wrong with Lindsey. I guess it was just another tantrum."

I have been asked about when I first heard that Lindsey had autism and how I felt. No one really told me that she had autism. I just kept on hearing the word. My mom was talking about it. My grandparents were talking about it. It seemed like everyone was talking about it. Autism...autism...autism...It was everywhere. For me, autism meant something really BAD! For me, autism meant something scary. For me, autism meant something sad. We were rarely happy because we were always thinking about autism.

This was my life, and I didn't know any other way. I didn't see any other kids like Lindsey, so I figured that no other families were dealing with the same things we were.

One day, I heard my mom crying in her bedroom. I slowly opened the door and saw her sitting on the bed. The green walls surrounded her, and the lights were dim. I sat by mom and started rubbing her back. I was a little girl just wanting my mom to be happy. I had so much I wanted to tell her and ask, but I didn't know how.

I wanted to ask, "Is Lindsey going to be like this forever?"

I wanted to ask, "Is our family going to be like Al's family someday?" Al was my best friend, and his family seemed happy all of the time. I also looked at my other cousins and their families, and they seemed to have so much fun with their siblings. Instead of doctor appointments, they were probably going to a park or watching movies in a theater.

In the months that followed, I remember going to many doctor appointments, and quite honestly, you can only play with that roller coaster toy for so long. When I would ask, "Can we leave now?" the response was either "In a few minutes," or "Hang in there." The few minutes typically turned into hours and hours.

When you get on a roller coaster, there is this feeling of anticipation. How fast will it go? How many twists and turns will there be? Will I get sick? Will I love it? All you do know is once you're strapped in, you are along for the ride. I learned early on that I would always be a part of my sister's rollercoaster.

Chapter Seven

"The stories of my early years give me mixed feelings."

By Lindsey Moreland

Throughout my younger years and my thoughts with having autism, I kept it a secret in my head. If I didn't talk about it, then maybe people wouldn't know about it. Today, I do not like watching the home videos of me screaming. Just last week, when we were working on the book over at my grandmother's house, my mom put in a home video because she wanted to do some research for the book. It made me anxious. I felt like bolting out of the house and tried my best to stay seated at the kitchen table. However, after 15-20 minutes, I couldn't watch it, and I ended up going outside. I walked around. I sat on a bench. I felt like crying. I was also getting uncomfortable listening to all of the stories. My family knew enough to leave me alone for a while and give me some time and space.

It makes me sad to think I put my family through so much when I was little. I'm relieved that I don't have memories of acting this way. I have memories of growing up, which you will read about later, but I do not have memories of the temper tantrums my parents talk about.

My decision to start talking about my autism has been inspired by several different events. It was the fall of 2010, and I was 16 ½ years old. My Grandma Moreland brought us a DVD of the movie Temple Grandin. I watched the whole movie, and after seeing that movie I was very teary. It brought back memories of how I behaved. Temple Grandin is an adult with autism. She has a PHD in animal science and has written several books. A year later, I went to the University of Wisconsin, River Falls and listened to Temple Grandin speak. With my mom by my side, I was somehow brave enough to walk up to her to meet her. I introduced myself, and I said, "I have autism." She seemed pleased that I mentioned it. For the first time in my life, I was able to say it out loud.

I was determined to find the courage to begin talking about autism. I was determined to help others to understand that it is ok to be different and to accept who you are as an individual. The stories of my early years give me mixed feelings. Sometimes I am proud that I am allowing others share stories about my growing-up-years. Other times it makes me sad.

Chapter Eight

"For me, autism is just a word."

By Todd Moreland, Lindsey's dad

In Iowa, we lived two blocks from the lake. We liked to take family walks to the lake. Lindsey and Brittany both loved the water. It had a nice sandy beach with a small park near it with swings, a jungle gym, and a backhoe shovel for digging in the sand. One Sunday afternoon, we took our family walk to the lake. It was time to leave, and Lindsey, in my words, "Blew a nut!" She threw herself to the ground and started banging her head screaming. It felt like forever. In fact, it didn't stop. I picked her up, and she screamed and kicked all the way home.

I was shocked that she was acting this way. I had never seen anything like it from her. I felt blindsided.

"Is there something truly wrong with Lindsey?" I wondered. I wished she could just talk to us instead of scream. The rest of it was all a blur. I have been asked if this is when I thought that I knew that she had autism. Quite honestly, I don't remember what I was thinking or feeling other than that I just wanted my little girl to stop crying.

I remember taking her into stores and the way other people would look at her. It made me furious. One time an older woman boldly stated, "Oh…ain't she a fussy one?" Lindsey was screaming. We didn't know why. Could we have gone down the wrong aisle? Could she have wanted something, and we didn't even know what she wanted? We were just trying to get what we needed and to get out of there. My thoughts were, "How dare you judge my kid?" Yet, I bit my lip and left as fast as I could.

For me, autism is just a word. It doesn't describe who my Lindsey was or is today. Regardless of the temper tantrums or the things that Lauri told me about Lindsey and autism in these early months and years, I choose to remember what I could do for her at her young age.

When Lindsey started watching Disney movies, I sat with her. It was an hour and half of no screaming. I soon knew every line to every movie that we watched. We watched them at least fifty times. Whenever we were at the store, we looked at the movies, often bought one, and quickly our family had an extensive selection of Disney movies. When I played with her, I would help her reenact the movies. She didn't smile much back then, but somehow I knew it made her happy.

The tantrum at the lake didn't stop us from taking her there. She loved the water, and I liked watching her play in it. I knew that someday I would buy a boat and hoped my two girls would go out and spend time with me in the boat. It was another reason to continue to work hard and provide for my family.

Because Lindsey loved bubbles and water, we did whatever it took to let her enjoy them. I spent time with her playing in the basement with the little kitchen set and let her blow bubbles all over the house. We would put her in the kitchen sink and let the water run. It didn't matter that it was all going down the drain or what the water bill for the month would cost. A home video of it shows her feeling the water as it comes out of the faucet. The water was her connection to the world when it felt like she had very little or no connection to us.

Shortly after, Lauri and I made the decision to move back to Wisconsin, and I began looking for a job. The only thing that was holding us there was my current job, but we both knew we needed and wanted more support for Lindsey.

Chapter Nine

"My parents said they should've bought stock in Disney"

By Lindsey Moreland

I have heard a lot of stories about how I acted when I was younger, before I remember hearing the word autism. Some of them I am not sure if I have remembered on my own, have seen on home videos, or remember because they were told to me over and over. Here are a few that I do remember.

My mom always said that toys frustrated me. I liked playing bubbles, but I didn't like when I couldn't hold the wand, and it didn't work right. Building blocks just fell down and would never stay up the way I wanted them. When I put my toys in a perfect line, my sister Brittany would come and take one out. The little red car in the basement was fun when the door would open and close on the first try, but not any other time. Our little pretend kitchen was equally fun unless a piece of food accidentally fell on the floor or someone wanted to share.

Thus, movies were my favorite way to spend my time. Movies were predictable, and that was what I liked. They never changed. They had the same beginning, middle, and end, including the previews and the credits. I watched movies every day, and if I had my way, all day.

My parents said they should have bought stock in Disney because my favorites were *Snow White, Sleeping Beauty, Aladdin*, and *Beauty and the Beast*. Although I didn't talk much, I could repeat lines from the movies, jump around, and hand flap in excitement.

Can you guess which movies these lines come from?

"Don't eat the apple." (*Snow White*)

"Don't touch the spinning wheel." (*Sleeping Beauty*)

"A Whole New World." (*Aladdin*)

"Be our Guest" (*Beauty and the Beast*)

"Khan, trust in me." (*The Jungle Book*)

My dad says that one of my favorites that I watched over and over was *The Jungle Book.*

My sister Brittany liked to watch the movies with me. It was the one thing we could do together when I was little. We liked to reenact scenes from the movies. We both liked to be the princesses, and that's when the fighting would start. I remember getting mad at her because she always seemed to get the character she wanted which was the princess. I was stuck being the prince or any other guy character. I was mad, but I acted it out anyway. It was predictable and safe for me. It was much better than any toy or person.

Chapter Ten

"It's Lindsey's way or the highway."

By Brittany Moreland, Lindsey's Sister

"Let's play *Barbies*!" I would say to Lindsey when she was little. She couldn't talk, so she would just throw the Barbie and spin around in circles. I wanted to make her happy because when she was happy she wasn't screaming. NO SCREAMING meant a peaceful, happy family. I always thought, "It is Lindsey's way or the highway."

My mom says that before Lindsey was born, I wasn't the best sharer either. When I was in daycare, they would ask if I was an only child, which I was. I guess I had a lot to learn about sharing, but when you grow up with a sibling with autism, you definitely learn to share quickly.

Whether one day I decided to make Lindsey's world happier, or it just happened subconsciously, I began doing things for Lindsey that would make her smile or laugh. I made up a spinning contest where we would spin together around and around until we would fall down. She would laugh. I felt like I was doing something right for her.

Often, I let her choose what we would play and which movie we would watch. We would start out liking the same movie. However, Lindsey would like it for a month. I could only handle it for about a week. Over time, Lindsey began to trust me and really see me as her friend, not just her sister. I wanted to be like her security blanket. I wanted to always "have her back." As Lindsey began to trust me more, I started to take advantage of her trust like any older sibling would do.

She would get to pick the movie we would reenact which always happened to be the movie of the month. Then, I would tell her that I got to be the princess. I guess we learned to give and take.

Years later when Lindsey did learn to talk, I would still act out movies with her to make her happy. It also seemed to be helping her speech. One day we were playing parts from *101 Dalmations*. Lindsey grabbed a straw and started to pretend to smoke like Cruella Deville.

My mom asked, "Lindsey, what are you doing?"

"I am smoking like Cruella Deville," Lindsey responded.

My mom told her that smoking was bad for her and naughty.

Lindsey was upset, "I am sorry. I am sorry. I will never do it again." This was the beginning of Lindsey's endless rules to follow because…It was Lindsey's way or the highway.

Chapter Eleven

"If I didn't have hope, at least I had help."

By Lauri Moreland, Lindsey's mom

"How is our family going to handle all of this?" I wondered.

Why can't I go to work and Todd stay home? Maybe then, he would see what I see. Maybe then, he would feel what I feel, and maybe then, he would hear what I hear. Todd has always been a man of few words. Yet, I felt like all of this was unfair. He never complained about working so many hours. I knew he wanted to try and fix everything for us because he would often say, "Just tell me what you want me to do." Still, I felt like it was unfair to be stuck at home every day with Lindsey screaming while trying to take care of other children. Putting on a happy face and trying extra hard to love these children became more challenging by the day.

Yet, every time I tried to talk to Todd about it, it felt like he blocked me out. I felt ignored and unheard. I wanted him to wrap his arms around me, hug me, and tell me that it was all going to be ok.

Todd shared the incident at the lake and the day that he realized there could possibly be some truth to what I had been trying to tell him for months. My recollection of the "Lake Story" is not the same as Todd's. Our differences are only in the details of the day, not the temper tantrum. My memory of that day includes a car ride to the lake. We wanted to spend time with the girls that didn't include a store or any other place where people would stare at us and judge us for being bad parents.

The temper tantrum is as clear in my mind today as it was 22 years ago. I, too remember the temper tantrum lasting forever. However, I recall a screaming drive home versus a walk. The temper tantrum didn't stop at home. It continued as she banged her head on the concrete driveway. While I was worried about her hurting herself, I was also embarrassed by the looks from all of the people outside that evening enjoying the lake. I could feel the world staring at us and judging us. A part of me was relieved, though, because Todd was finally seeing my everyday life with Lindsey. Interestingly enough, my mom's version of the lake story is most similar to Todd's which again is a reminder that our memories belong to us but often differ from others involved.

My classmate Susan, who continued to be concerned with our situation, called again for an update. She asked, "What is keeping you in Iowa?"

I responded, "This house…I guess, nothing." After more phone calls and visits from friends and family, it was evident to Todd and me that the best decision would be to move back to Wisconsin, closer to our family support system. We were fortunate to not only have my parents' support us from afar, but also guide us in our decision to move back. My Uncle Jerome helped Todd find a job in Minnesota about 40 minutes from Wisconsin. My Aunt Marcella let us know that she would be available to help with Lindsey, too. Her famous words were, "Remember, I am a professional volunteer." In addition to these people we would also be living near my four siblings, their spouses and their young children. I have many aunts, uncles & cousins living in Wisconsin that had already offered to help our family.

It seems surreal now, and I am not sure how I would ever be able to repay all of the family and friends that helped us move back to Wisconsin, yet I can remember my cousin Mike showing up in the driveway with a semi ready to help us move. As I watched my siblings, my parents, other relatives, and friends load up all of our belongings, for an instant I had hope. If I didn't have hope, at least I had help.

Chapter Twelve

"I was moving away from my best friend."

By Brittany Moreland, Lindsey's sister

Even though my family was going through so much while living in Iowa, my memories are of the fun times. I had a best friend named Al. We did everything together including preschool, watching the show *Gargoyles*, and having sleepovers. My mom did daycare for Al and his sister Kay. He was the one person that made me forget about autism. When Lindsey banged her head on the brick wall, I knew something was going to change, but I didn't expect that change was moving away from my best friend.

I remember helping my family get things out of the moving truck at our new home in Wisconsin.

I turned to my mom and said, "I miss Al already." I thought to myself, "Why did I have to move away from him?"

My mom replied, "I know, but it will get better."

As sad as I was, I knew the bright side was that my cousins were living downstairs in the duplex in which we were living. Years and years later, I found Al on Facebook, and we both laughed at all the memories we shared.

Living in Wisconsin was a big change. The only thing that I was happy about was that I was living closer to my grandparents and cousins on my mom's side. I didn't like the school I attended. I felt that some of the teachers were mean to me. Plus, I had a learning disability that made school really difficult. I struggled with both reading and math. Nothing seemed fair. While I was at school, Lindsey would go to a special children's center in a town nearby. The center looked like it was so much fun, but it was always for Lindsey, not for me. Therapists would praise her, swing her, and she got to go swimming a lot.

Some days instead of going back to our apartment or waiting at the center, my mom and I would go to great grandma's house. We would drive up a dirt road to her "cottage" which was on my great uncle's farm. It was really a trailer house, but it was fancy and Great Grandma was proud of it, so she called it her "cottage." We would eat homemade sugar cookies, play card games like *Go Fish*, listen to the ocean with her sea shells, and if I was lucky I would get to play the organ alongside my mom and Great Grandma. Not everyone was lucky enough to get to play the organ. It was Great Grandma's pride and joy. I was so happy and thankful. For a couple hours a week, it felt like "Brittany Time." I also appreciated when the therapist would let me do a swimming day at the center with Lindsey.

When I was about 5 years old, I qualified to go to the center due to Hip Click which was a condition that was inhibiting my ability to walk properly. I was with the same therapist Lindsey had, and I got pictures taken like Lindsey. For a minute, I felt I was getting the same attention as Lindsey. Even though Lindsey threw a lot of tantrums, I still wanted to be by her.

When Lindsey was enrolled in Early Childhood, she had to go to school, too. However, she had to ride a special education bus. I begged my mom for us to ride the same bus. I got to one day. We had seatbelts on the bus, but mine was not working. I was sitting by another child with autism. I assumed she was like Lindsey and didn't want to be touched. So, I left more space between us than I normally would.   The bus driver was a fast driver. Let's just say, after that, I rode my old bus again.

The one thing I looked forward to was hanging out with my cousins. Things were not great, but it seemed to be getting a little better. We had been living in Wisconsin for three years. My parents decided Lindsey needed more help. Along with this decision, another move was being talked about.

Chapter Thirteen

"It's not autism yet."

By Lauri Moreland, Lindsey's Mom

Moving back to Wisconsin gave me a glimpse of peace and hope, but with it came many changes. The changes were beyond what others could see or what I wanted to show. It wasn't that we were moving from a three bedroom home with three living rooms, two kitchens, and a screened in porch in a good neighborhood that bothered me. It wasn't that we now only had a two bedroom apartment, small kitchen and small living room, either. In fact, a stranger looking at us would have thought we were a perfectly functional family. It was quite the contrary.

Lindsey's behavior, including the tantrums continued. The medical part of dealing with autism was taking its toll on me. Prior to moving back to Wisconsin, Lindsey had a MRI. The MRI came back normal. However, with the possible Pervasive Developmental Disorder, early intervention services were recommended in Iowa. My high school classmate Susan suggested we contact Birth to Three in Wisconsin right away. After contacting them and many phone calls later, two therapists came to the apartment. Lindsey was 2 years, 3 months old. The reports state that Lindsey was functioning at an approximate twelve month developmental level. In addition, she was unresponsive with certain language communication skills. Again, a hearing evaluation was done and that came out normal.

Meanwhile, I was dealing with SSI (Social Security Income). We felt misled by the insistence to apply for the money. I don't remember how much it even was each month. While it was helpful, we soon found out that they were asking for it all back. We didn't have the energy to look for a new house in Wisconsin when we were trying to help Lindsey. Instead of buying a new house, we took some of the money from the sale of our home in Iowa and bought land thinking we would build on it someday. It soon came to our attention that we had too many assets even though I was consistent and honest on my monthly reports. I felt like I was on trial. I was even reporting antiques I had in my house that had been given to me from my grandma. I remember specific conversations where the operator was drilling me on the antiques that I was never planning to sell anyway. It was another nightmare. A court appearance was scheduled, and I was confident that I could prove that we were using the money properly. Unfortunately, it didn't matter. Our move and the assets from it required us to pay all of the money back. To this day, it doesn't make sense to me and felt like an added burden on our family.

Luckily, my brother Dennis and sister-in-law Nancy, who owned the duplex where we were living, lived in the lower level. They were amazing to us and a huge support. I am certain that if we had not been living with them at the time and had to live somewhere else, we would have been evicted multiple times due to Lindsey's screaming and tantrums. They knew when we were having a bad day, which was every day. Not only did they give us the space we needed when we needed it, they were also available anytime we asked. It confirmed my belief that my house and the space we left was not important. We had family and a place to live.

Now that we were living in Wisconsin, my classmate Susan became my friend. She was there for me every single day. We talked and went on walks whenever we could. She taught me how to be an advocate for Lindsey and my family. She guided me towards the available services. Susan was living her own story with autism. Susan's daughter was diagnosed with autism approximately a year before our concerns with Lindsey began. Her family was working extremely hard to help their daughter and implemented multiple different therapies and services. Here she was going through her own hell and yet she had become my lifeline to getting Lindsey the help she needed.

Upon meeting with therapists, I felt the need for a second opinion and more thorough evaluation. In my mind, Lindsey didn't have autism just yet or perhaps they made a mistake in the diagnosis. The letter said, "Possible Pervasive Developmental Disorder." It did NOT say autism! Much of what you have read so far in this book has included us declaring or thinking that Lindsey had been officially diagnosed with autism in Iowa. As a parent of a child with autism, there is a lot of denial, and even though that word has been said so often, in my mind at this particular time, it was NOT absolute.

Susan, along with Pediatric Therapy Services in Wisconsin gave me the name of a renowned psychologist named Lyle Chastain. They also put in a referral for Lindsey to be further evaluated by Lyle Chastain. With all of Lindsey's needs, I was learning how to become a better advocate for her. I called Lyle Chastain's office and talked with her secretary. My biggest concern was trying to get Lindsey into the office to see Lyle Chastain. I told the secretary, "Lindsey will not even walk over the threshold of the door." I had plenty of evidence to back this up. Whenever we took Lindsey to a new place, she flipped out on us. She would fall to the ground, bang her head, cry, and scream. In addition, she did not want people to look at her or touch her. I felt like she was just really afraid. After explaining the situation, the secretary told me that this was not uncommon with other children. I was so relieved when she said Lyle Chastain could come to our apartment, Lindsey's own environment. At the time I had no idea Ms. Chastain was known nationally and internationally as a pioneer in the field of autism.

She helped to start the Fraser Autism Center of Excellence.

Fraser Autism Center of Excellence

Minneapolis, MN

612-861-1688

www.Fraser.org

Chapter Fourteen

"I was going to build a swing set fit for my princesses."

By Todd Moreland, Lindsey's dad

Our Iowa house was only on the market for four days. It happened so fast. At that time, I had heard the word autism, but it needed to be confirmed or diagnosed by a specialist before Lindsey could get some outside help.

After Lindsey was officially labeled with autism, I continued to look for things that I could give her to help her find some happiness in this world.

Speech and occupational therapists began coming to our apartment to work with Lindsey. They were also helping her learn how to socialize. I felt like Lindsey and Brittany needed something to play with outside. Lindsey loved swinging, and it was often part of her therapy. I told Lauri I wanted to go to Menards and look at swing sets. My brother-in-law was happy to have us build a swing set in the back yard because they had two small children as well. After deciding which swing set we wanted to build and over $1,000 dollars later, I was going to build a swing set fit for my princesses. I wanted the best for my girls, and I spent hours looking through lumber at Menards finding the best, most perfect pieces.

The swing set took three days for my brother-in-law Dennis and me to build. It had a tower, a climbing rope, a slide, four swings, and a sandbox. It was my way of doing anything I could to help not only Lindsey, but also Brittany as we continued to survive living with autism. All of a sudden, the swing set became the neighborhood "hot spot" for kids. Lindsey didn't always like this because she didn't like being around other people, especially ones she didn't know. The therapists were pleased with the swing set and would often use it during her in-home therapy.

Chapter Fifteen

"The label made it official."

By Ida Feyereisen, Lindsey's grandma

I was fussing over a chicken casserole that I had offered to make for lunch and was upset when it boiled over and messed up Lauri's oven. It smelled bad, yet didn't seem like it was done in the middle. Why would I even consider making something new for this day? Why was it such a big deal to me? Lauri and Todd were dealing with something monumental in our lives, and I was fretting over food.

Since Todd was at a new job with no available time off, Lauri asked if I could come and be with her at their new apartment in Wisconsin. Lyle Chastain was coming to evaluate Lindsey. When she arrived, I immediately sensed that she was a gentle, sweet lady. After she had observed Lindsey for a short time, I got the feeling that she already knew what her diagnosis would be. However, it wasn't like going to the clinic for blood work and waiting for results. At one point during her visit Lindsey was watching the movie *101 Dalmatians*. As the star in the movie was playing the piano, Lindsey went to their piano and ran her fingers over the covered keyboard area and pretended to play. I knew it was a good sign, and I wanted to run up and hug her and tell her how smart she was, but of course I knew that would upset her. Ms. Chastain's house call lasted several hours, but her official diagnosis didn't come until the end of her visit.

At 28 months, Lindsey displayed significant, undeniable symptoms of a child with autism. The label was official. Lindsey Moreland was a child with autism. That day was extremely devastating and especially hard on Lauri as Ms. Chastain confirmed what Lauri so desperately hoped would not be true.

Some labels are harsh, and being told that your child has been labeled with any form of physical, mental, psychological delay, or serious illness is heart wrenching. But as I see it, in today's world, without that label, the essential help that parents need is not readily available. I didn't realize it at the time, but I believe the label made a world of difference in the very special person Lindsey has become.

* Lyle Chastain of Minneapolis, Minnesota died of cancer on Oct 14, 2013, according to her obituary in the Minneapolis Star Tribune.

Chapter Sixteen

"There are no ANDs...IFs... or BUTs....Lindsey has autism."

By Lauri Moreland, Lindsey's Mom

May 13, 1996, I told Todd to go to work. It was going to be a busy day in our little apartment. Brittany was spending the day with my sister Linda and her kids. My mom, Lyle Chastain, Lindsey's speech therapist, her occupational therapist, and a social worker would all be attending "THE meeting," which was a second, and final, opinion with regards to a diagnosis for Lindsey. Lindsey had been working with therapists since we had moved back to Wisconsin through the Birth to Three Program. I had done all of the necessary paperwork back when we lived in Iowa so that this could be started right away. The word autism was brought up over and over by therapists, family, and friends...but always with the disclaimer, "I am not in the position to verify it." Upon the suggestion of Susan and the therapists, Lyle Chastain was contacted.

As I replay the day in my mind, I continue to have butterflies in my stomach. I can't believe that I told Todd to go to work on one of the most important days of our family's life. I didn't want Ms. Chastain, a psychologist, to say the word "autism," OR did I want her to say it? Inside I was struggling. Did Lindsey REALLY have autism or could it possibly be something else? Everything I read pointed in that direction. There was nothing good about it. I remember feeling like a bad mom. I remember reading that children with autism end up living in institutions. I remember reading that most people with autism don't end up talking or aren't even capable of being toilet trained. Sadly, I focused on every negative piece of information out there. Honestly, in my opinion, over twenty years ago, there wasn't anything positive to read about autism. It felt like it was a death sentence.

Lyle Chastain's visit lasted over four hours. In that time, she observed Lindsey pulling me around the apartment. If Lindsey wanted something, she would push me into a room. She would expect me to know what she wanted. If I picked the wrong thing, it caused a tantrum. At times, she pushed my hand into the object that she desired. It was obvious to everyone that I was being used as a tool to get what Lindsey needed or wanted.

Ms. Chastain had us bring out different toys. As we sat on the floor trying to play with Lindsey, Lyle observed Lindsey's lack of interaction with us. Lindsey was spinning, flapping, screaming, and did not make eye contact. Furthermore, she became upset when we changed toys or brought out different toys. It was impossible to keep Lindsey engaged with an activity. She wandered the apartment looking confused. Moving on from the toys, we put in a video for Lindsey to watch. Ms. Chastain instructed us to follow along with the movie and try to get Lindsey to copy us. She encouraged Lindsey to use the movie language instead of screaming.

At one point, Lindsey pulled me into the kitchen and started screaming. I frantically pulled out several food items such as boxes of cereal, crackers, and chips. Trying to find what she wanted, I became even more frustrated as she continued to scream. This was my everyday life and now Lyle Chastain, a highly recommended psychologist specializing in autism, was witnessing it. I could have been embarrassed, but I wasn't. Lindsey's therapists and my mom were used to seeing how she acted. Yet, it was a defining moment for me because my world was being exposed at a whole new level. There was no denying what they saw.

Lyle interrupted my interactions with Lindsey. Although soft spoken, Ms. Chastain made it clear to us we could not continue living like this. Lindsey was controlling the household. The louder she screamed, the faster we all moved. Ms. Chastain introduced Mayer Johnson symbols, which are picture communication symbols. The example she gave to us was milk. The symbol for milk was on a 2 by 2 inch card and put on the refrigerator. We were to teach Lindsey to hand us the symbol card as we said the word. The goal was for her to eventually say the word as she handed us the symbol.

Throughout the meeting, Lyle Chastain continued instructing the therapists on what we should be working on to help Lindsey progress. As Ms. Chastain was giving us pointers on how to help her, I didn't even wonder if we would get an official diagnosis that day. I was used to going to the doctor and waiting for test results to be returned in a week or more. After four hours of observations and working with us, I asked Ms. Chastain, "When do we find out if Lindsey has autism?"

Her response was, "I was waiting for you to ask." She continued, "I hate this part of my job. There are no ANDs...IFs...or BUTs....Lindsey has autism."

Instantly, I began to cry. Ms. Chastain told me that she was sorry. Through the tears and the numbness throughout my body, I heard the words, "Time is on our side...and you have no time to waste."

My mom hugged me. Soon after, everyone, including my mom, packed up their things and left. I quickly called Susan and told her the official news of the diagnosis. Continuing to cry, I put Lindsey in her car seat and drove to my sister's house to pick up Brittany. When I got to my sister's house, I told her that Lindsey had autism. Her response was devastating to me as she said, "Didn't you already know that?"

On the way home, I couldn't believe how unsurprised everyone else was. They acted as if it was just another day. For me, the months of waiting for a final diagnosis was here. I was hoping for compassionate responses and understanding rather than the matter of fact reactions I received. When I came home, there was a beautiful bouquet of flowers with a card on my table. It was from Susan.

The card said, "I am here for you." Susan understood.

When Todd walked in the door after work, I told him that Lindsey had autism. There was no response. He never said the word autism for about a year. Once again I felt so alone. I knew he cared, but he just couldn't talk about it.

Chapter Seventeen
We all screamed, "STOP!"
By Todd Moreland, Lindsey's Dad
Title Named by Lindsey

I went to work at a truck utilities company in Minnesota, which was about a half hour drive away from our apartment. It was May 13, 1996, (Lindsey provided this date for me) and it was like any other work day. When I got home, Lauri told me that Lyle Chastain diagnosed Lindsey with autism. Other than that, I don't remember anything else about that day. Yes, it was a diagnosis, but it wasn't going to change anything for me or how she was acting. It also wouldn't change how much I loved her or how I would try to parent her. I didn't even know what autism was, and because I was working "all these hours" trying to support our family, it was just one more thing to deal with. I wanted to move forward. However, after that, I do remember how Lindsey began to communicate with us.

Lindsey was being taught sign language through therapy and was also being taught how to use pictures to communicate with us. The pictures were little cards and symbols. We kept them in a three ring binder. For example, there was a food card, drink card, and a book. There was also one that I remember of a coat and a kid going outside. The one she brought to me most was the movie card. She also got really good at the sign for "milk" and "more." She drank milk 24-7, so we all got good at that sign.

Lindsey and I spent a lot of time out on the playground I built. Part of her therapy was swinging. I would swing her to calm her down. The best part is that she would smile and laugh.

As I am telling this story, I couldn't remember when exactly I got our family boat, so I asked Lindsey. Right away she said, "1996 in early spring or early summer." I had wanted to get a boat for our family. I knew how much Lindsey loved water, and I also liked fishing. When I started looking for boats, I looked at a used boat about a block away from our house. I asked the guy selling it, "Does it leak?"

His response was, "Not really." He was asking $500. I was not impressed. I did not want a boat that might be unsafe for my family. The same day I drove to a nearby boat store. After looking around, I called Lauri to tell her I found a used one and wanted her to come and look at it, but I left that day the proud owner of a new boat and couldn't wait to take Lindsey, Brittany, and Lauri out on the water. I wondered if Lindsey would like it as much as I hoped she would.

My mom and dad came to visit us from Iowa soon after. We decided to take the boat out on a lake that wasn't far from our apartment. We spent a couple hours out on the lake because the weather was beautiful. When we were done and were putting the boat onto the trailer, I noticed Lindsey was in a dead bolt running towards the lake. We all screamed, "STOP!" Lauri was freaking out!

There was no stopping her; she jumped right into the lake, wanting to get back into the water. It was a good thing that she had her life jacket on because the water was deep. Lindsey floated around in her life jacket and there was no point trying to change her mind. We waited and waited and kind of just let her do her thing. She finally got tired of it and was ready to get out.

With Lindsey, we learned to allow her to do what she needed to do as long as she was safe. This is what it was like parenting Lindsey in those early years. If it wasn't hurting anyone else and we had the time for it, we allowed Lindsey to experience life the way it made sense to her. The one thing that I did intervene on and had enough of was her wearing a diaper at four years old. When Lindsey was four years old, Lauri convinced me to go to a family autism support group. It was a Christmas party. When we got there, I was shocked at how out of control all of the children were. The other parents seemed oblivious to all of it. I watched a parent change their 12 year old child's diaper, and it really bothered me. We didn't stay long because it was too chaotic for Lindsey and me. In the car ride home, I told Lauri, "I am not going to be changing my 12 year old daughter's diaper." It took until the following Easter to get Lindsey to begin the potty training process.

I told Lindsey, "We are not going to Grandma and Grandpa's until you go potty on the toilet." Three hours later, she went. Lauri and Brittany were not happy that they were missing out on family time including an Easter dinner, a jam session in the music room, and an egg hunt, but I was determined to get Lindsey potty trained. After she went to the bathroom, we attended the family gathering. Grandma Ida made sure to hide a few eggs for Brittany to have her own egg hunt. The family was supportive which we appreciated. Within days, she was completely trained. I will never regret the decision I made that day. Lindsey loved going to grandma's house, and it motivated her in this situation.

Chapter Eighteen

"Mayer Johnson Symbols"

By Ida Feyereisen, Lindsey's Grandma

Before Lindsey started to talk, Lauri came to our house with several sheets of Mayer Johnson Symbols printed on sheets of copy paper. Each sheet contained several rows of 2 inch square black and white pictures. They were simple and all different. Lauri explained that Lyle Chastain and the therapists hoped that these symbols would help Lindsey communicate. We sat at the picnic table in our backyard and cut the symbols apart as Lindsey played in the sandbox and on the swings. The symbols I remember that helped Lindsey the most at our house were: car, eat, water, swing, and milk. We put these small symbols on our refrigerator, and Lindsey soon learned to go to the refrigerator and point to, or bring us the symbol that indicated what she wanted. Everyone was excited the first time she brought us the picture of the glass of milk. It sure beat watching her stand in the middle of the floor (not even close to the refrigerator) screaming.

Along with the Mayer Johnson Symbols, Lindsey was learning sign language. Sadly, some children with autism never become verbal, so there was always the possibility that Lindsey would never talk. In that case, we hoped she could learn to sign. Her therapists' plans were always for her to learn to say a word as she signed it, and to eventually no longer need to sign. How excited we were when she said "more" as she signed it when she wanted more milk! The excitement grew as she eventually said "more" as she signed the word each time she wanted another push on the swing. We praised her and praised her, and she laughed and laughed. It was very evident that she was so pleased with herself.

Lauri didn't always have someone to leave the girls with when she wanted or needed to go somewhere. She wanted so badly to take the girls with her like most mothers could without incident. One day she asked me to go with her and the girls to *Wal-Mart*. She had already had some bad experiences in stores and wanted me there for support. As soon as we got inside the building, Lindsey threw herself down on the floor and began kicking and screaming. Customers and staff stared at us. I can only imagine what they were thinking. They looked at us as if Lindsey was naughty and uncontrollable. We knew there was no way she could tell us what was bothering her. You can't blame the bystanders, they didn't understand. The word "autism" was so new to most of us at that time.

After this incident, I decided to see if a picture (like the Mayer Johnson Symbols) of the Wal-Mart store might help. By this time we had learned that showing Lindsey a picture of where you were going made the car ride more pleasant. So, I called the manager of the local Wal-Mart and asked if I could come and take a picture of the parking lot, the outside of the front of the store, and some inside the store showing things like toys that Lindsey might be interested in seeing. It took some explaining about autism and how I felt this might help Lindsey. The manager said I could take a photo of the parking lot and the outside front of the store, but I would have to come in and ask for him before I could take pictures inside. He looked at my camera and must have been convinced that neither the inexpensive camera nor I looked professional enough to be a spy. However, I was only allowed to stand a few feet into the store with him by my side as I snapped a few pictures. I was not allowed to take pictures of the toy aisle, but that might have been good because I seem to remember it was difficult to get her away from the toy department in the years that followed. I believe the pictures were useful to help her understand where she was going. It took a long time for her to become comfortable inside the store. Maybe the lights, sounds, crowds, or something unknown even to her made her uncomfortable.

"Mayer-Johnson" 1 (800) 588 – 4548

mjq@tobiidynavox.com

PO Box 72153, Cleveland, OH 44192

Chapter Nineteen

"Love is patient."

By Lauri Moreland, Lindsey's mom

Soon after Lindsey's diagnosis, it was apparent that we lived in a home with a revolving door. I would have loved to have a day where I never got out of my pajamas or never worried about if my house was clean enough. Instead, I was always worried about appearances. Therapists came to our apartment three times each week. We had home visits with social workers, teachers, and meetings about respite care. Because of what we had gone through with SSI, Social Security Income, I felt like our family was always being watched, like a bug under a microscope.

On top of all of the home visits, I drove Lindsey to a special children's center three times each week. When Lindsey was with other people, I often wondered how she would be treated or how she would get what she needed.

Would she hurt someone or herself during a tantrum?

Would she eat anything or starve herself?

Would she need me or not even care?

I loved Lindsey so much, yet it took every ounce of me to never lay a hand on her. My inner being wanted to spank her or shake her when a tantrum overtook the day.

However, I knew that was not the answer, and it would only make it worse while alienating any chance of a relationship with her. I was her mother and needed as much patience as possible to get through each day. If I had these feelings, how could the therapists and teachers stay patient enough to not harm her? If they ever did, how could she ever tell me what happened? Even my own grandmother questioned me about Lindsey's behavior...and why couldn't we just give her an old-fashioned spanking?

Chapter Twenty

"I know what those kids need..."

By Ida and Steve Feyereisen, Lindsey's grandparents

Lindsey's Grandpa Steve, now in his early eighties, recently spent a typical Thursday afternoon visiting with other neighborhood men in the shop on his brother's farm. Because the farm is up the road from our house, one of the men asked, "What are the extra cars doing in your yard today?"

Grandpa Steve explained that it was his two daughters and granddaughter Lindsey. They were working on writing a book about Lindsey's life with autism. The neighborhood man asked, "What is autism?"

Grandpa talked about Lindsey's early years with autism and how there were lots of behavioral problems including screaming, yelling, and head banging. The gentleman replied, "I know what those kids need...a good spanking!"

These are common misconceptions of children with autism. When it was first suggested that Lindsey might have autism, our knowledge of it was minimal. We had so much to learn. Would we ever be able to hold her, cuddle her, sing to her, love her, and have her return that love? Would we lose her forever to her own little world? Oh how we prayed, her Grandpa Steve and me, along with many friends and relatives. We knew the power of prayer, and at this time, there was little else we could do. Sure we loved her, and always would love her. No matter how hard everyone tried, no expression of love was accepted by Lindsey. It only seemed to make matters worse.

Throughout the years since Lindsey was born, Grandpa Steve and I have felt the need to not only defend Lindsey's behavior but that of other children that appear as just being "naughty." It is not as if our own five children were never disciplined. We held high expectations for respectful behavior both in our home and in public. When our children misbehaved, there were definitely consequences. However, as far as we are concerned, it is not a tiny baby's choice to be naughty. From the beginning of her life, Lindsey's behavior was different than any other child with which I had a connection.

I was proud to hear Grandpa Steve's response to the neighborhood friend. After 22 years, he was continuing to defend not only Lindsey, but all children with special needs.

"You have no idea what is going on with a screaming child in a store, a church, or any other public place," he answered very sternly. "It's possible that the parent is doing all they can for a child who might have autism. It's not the kid's fault either. They don't know how to make us understand what they want."

After reading this chapter to Grandpa, he not only approved it, he also said, "You've heard me get hot and frustrated before, well this time I was really hot!"

Chapter Twenty-One

"I CAN'T do this anymore!"

By Lauri Moreland, Lindsey's mom

In the months that followed, I continued to struggle emotionally and physically every day. All of it was draining me. Nothing in my world seemed fair. Our families, with good intentions, often gave us advice about praying more and rarely could see how difficult our family situation was for Todd, Brittany, Lindsey, and me. My father would tell me not to be angry with God (which I wasn't) and told me to go to church more to "Get the Word." What he didn't see, that consumed me, were the stares, the embarrassment when we had to get up and leave, and the hurtful words of others such as, "There is a cry room." Constantly, I felt judged. My memories of growing up going to church were happy and comfortable, but now church provided no comfort for me and it just added stress.

It wasn't just church that was uncomfortable and stressful. We couldn't go anywhere as a family without causing a huge scene. We couldn't go shopping. We couldn't go to a movie. We couldn't go to a park. We tried to attend family functions, but we were often the first to leave with tears and always in dramatic fashion. Lindsey couldn't handle changes in her routine. Even though I believed our family was understanding and not judging like the public was, it still hurt. More than anything, I wanted our family to be like any other family, normal.

One evening, I couldn't take it anymore. I drove to my parents' house by myself. Todd was watching the girls. I visited with my parents at the kitchen table for a short while. As I was getting ready to leave, I stopped at the door and burst into tears.

"I can't do this anymore," I cried. My next words were, "I think I am going to have to put Lindsey in an institution. She is wrecking my life, Brittany's life, and Todd's life...and she is NOT happy. She doesn't want to be here either."

My mom and dad hugged me and said they were here for me. They begged me to ask for more help and to not consider putting Lindsey in an institution. My mom even went so far as to say, "We will take her."

I replied, "Like that's going to work...that will be in the paper with the headlines reading, *Grandparents take child because Mother can't handle her.*"

I never told my parents about the many thoughts I had each time I drove to my part-time job as a hair stylist in Minnesota. I only worked 10-12 hours a week, but the drive there and back gave me lots of time to think about how I could end our current situation. I would dream up and visualize solutions. One of those visions included driving into the water that I passed each day with Lindsey in the car with me. I would try to make it look like an accident, and we could die together. In my mind, Todd and Brittany's life would be better. Lindsey would no longer have to suffer. I am not proud of this thinking, but it's real, and I know others who have family members with autism have had similar feelings. When you love someone so much and you feel helpless, you truly think there has to be a way to make life easier.

Chapter Twenty-Two

"I was doing what it takes to make everyone happy."

By Todd Moreland, Lindsey's dad

Lauri was not satisfied with the amount of help Lindsey was getting at school. She decided we should move to a different district that would offer Lindsey more support. Immediately I began looking for homes or land for building in the district Lauri chose. I saw an advertisement in the paper for a split level, model home. It was in a development in a small town, twenty miles away from our apartment. Lauri and I went to look at it. Deciding we liked it, we found land in the development, and built the new home. The builder built most of the house, but we put on a deck, stained the trim and doors, put in a yard, moved the swing set to the yard, and finished the basement to meet our needs. We designed the basement to accommodate Lindsey's therapy. There was room for a ball pit (6 ft. diameter), a trampoline, and a hammock swing. There was also a gigantic closet with shelves to organize all of Lindsey's things. A lot of it was her therapy toys and tools, but it was all organized for her in a way she could understand. We lived there for three and a half years.

Due to our staggered work schedules and the fact that our girls required more specialized care than what an after school program could offer, Lauri and I met at a ride share three times a week for two years. Here we said a brief hello, exchanged any important updates or information, and she handed over the girls to me so that she could get to work on time. During these years, I often took the girls out on the boat on a local lake. They invited cousins to join them. When the cousins came, I did very little fishing. I spent most of the time helping the kids. It was quite challenging, but everyone had fun. I started looking for land to buy near that lake. We wanted to move out of town and closer to the lake where we could make more great memories.

I saw an ad in the paper that interested me, for land near a lake, but it was two hours away. I asked if they had anything near what we considered to be "our lake" because we went there so much. I almost fell over when they said they did. It was four acres, and it was priced less than we expected. I felt like it was a deal we couldn't pass up. It was the exact piece of land that we wanted, so we bought it.

Once we had the land, we decided to build a log home. Lauri always dreamed of having a log home. With everything going on with Lindsey's autism and Brittany's epilepsy (more on that later), I hoped this would be a positive distraction and something to make her happy. I hoped. The building process did not go as planned. It took longer than expected, and the builder did not meet the agreed upon contract. In addition, a storm hit our house and caused extensive damage. We ended up having to fix pretty much everything including windows, roof, stonework, trim, and more. The maintenance alone on a log home is a lot of work. It is like a part time job. However, it was a beautiful home once it was finished.

Being closer to the lake was great. We bought the girls a paddle boat. Lindsey got a kayak. She loved kayaking on the lake. We also got a Collie puppy that looked just like Lassie. Brittany named the dog Buddy. Part of the reason we got a dog was for Brittany. We thought a dog would really help Brittany feel better about everything. She was sad and cried a lot. Maybe a dog would help. I wanted a Collie because of their reputation for being gentle and an all-around good dog.

Lindsey loved our dog Buddy, too. She liked to come with me when I took him to the nursing home to visit residents. Lindsey was obsessed with dates and liked to ask the residents how old they were. The residents were often proud to announce their age. She would quickly tell them the year they were born. If they told her their birthday, she could tell them the day of the week it was on as well. We all became dependent on Lindsey's great gift of memorizing dates, and we still depend on her today.

At the edge of our land, I built a treehouse for Lindsey. She went to her treehouse every day she could. Fortunately, for me, it also became a great tree stand for hunting.

As a father who sees his family struggling with medical conditions and the emotional effects from them, I was doing anything I could to try to make good memories for my girls and Lauri. I worked two jobs almost all of the time just to pay for things that I thought would help our family get through each day.

When your family is going through hard times, you have to have a way to escape thinking about it. It is not that you don't want to help or make it better, but sometimes you just can't make it better. My escapes were going out on the lake in the summer and ice fishing in the winter. I am also an avid hunter, and being in the woods is my tranquility. I took up bow hunting which gave me a lot of time in the woods by myself. When you get away for a few hours, there is nothing to bother you. Sitting in the woods for three hours for me is the perfect way to relax. I have gotten a lot of deer over the years. This put a lot of meat on the table and a few deer heads on the wall. The girls always refused to eat venison, so I told them it was beef. They ate it, and thought it was delicious. After three or four years, I broke down and told them they were eating venison. Their reaction at first was being mad, but later they admitted it was good. Hunting and fishing continue to be my escapes, but I also try to include the girls whenever they want to join me.

As a family that has children with special needs, Lauri and I made a commitment to support each other's interests and give each other time needed away from the daily stresses. When I would come home from work, Lauri would leave to go to the gym to exercise and have some time alone. She also supported my hunting and fishing. Lauri and I have been married 30 years. It's been a lot of give and take. When the girls were very young, we always did things as a family and took turns watching the girls whenever the other one needed a break because who would watch the girls? As the girls got older and were old enough to be left alone, Lauri and I could go out together. We have enjoyed listening to bands and watching movies. I am grateful that our family stayed together and survived all of the hard times.

Chapter Twenty-Three
"Lindsey goes to school."

By Lauri Moreland, Lindsey's mom

Todd talked about moving and building our home, but why? When we lived in our apartment, in addition to all of her therapy, Lindsey also went to early childhood classes through the public school system. I would walk my little three year old girl with autism to the end of our driveway each morning. A yellow school bus would approach and Lindsey would happily get on the bus to see her bus driver. She would sit in the same seat each day all by herself in an almost empty bus. She was the first stop, and her bus ride was about 20 minutes. She would get home each day by lunchtime, yet I worried every second she was gone. I wondered if she would eat the snack. I wondered how many temper tantrums she would have or how she would handle them changing her diaper.

Communication with her teachers consisted of a daily notebook and many phone calls. They tried to stay positive, but I could feel it wasn't going as well as we all hoped. In time, the teachers reported that some progress was being made. "Baby steps," I thought. In contrast, afternoons with Lindsey were difficult. She insisted on the same schedule each day. For example, if it was lightning outside and she couldn't go out to swing on her swing set, she would bang her head, kick the door, pull the handle, and scream at the top of her lungs. She couldn't understand why she couldn't go outside to swing, and nothing I said or did would convince her that she needed to stay inside. She would scream for hours or until she passed out from crying and exhaustion. She would wake up 5 minutes later, and it would all begin again.

The therapists suggested that I videotape her so that she could watch herself acting out. My heart ached as I videotaped her, but it was even worse when she saw herself because she cried and screamed. It was clear that she didn't want to behave the way she was behaving, but she could not communicate with me, and she could not handle day to day changes without throwing a fit. I knew that she needed more help even though she received early childhood, in home therapy, and therapy through a special children's center.

Part of me wanted to give up, but the words of Lyle Chastain were always being replayed in my head. Lyle Chastain said, "Time is on your side, and we have no time to waste." She also reaffirmed what I believed...that Lindsey needed more and more help. The more help the better. I trusted her advice because she had worked with children with autism for many years and saw evidence that early interventions made a significant difference. Even though much of Ms. Chastain's visit was a blur for me at the time, her words often drove me to fight for Lindsey's future. When Lindsey was having a bad temper tantrum, I would remind myself that Lyle Chastain said often the children that have the most temper tantrums are the ones that are fighters. She had said that they are the children that want to communicate but just haven't figured out how to **yet**. I know that this advice doesn't always work out for every child or family. However, it gave me hope, and hope is what I needed.

Lindsey's school teachers informed me that I would be receiving an invitation in the mail to attend her IEP (Individualized Education Plan) meeting. I had already been to her initial evaluation meeting, so this was to renew her plan. Even though these meetings can be extremely intimidating, I was looking forward to it and prepared to ask for more help. When you walk into a room and there are eight people sitting around the table all there for your child, you think about what they are going to say. You prepare yourself for what you might hear. I was not prepared to hear that she was the most challenging student they had at the time. I was also not prepared for them to say, "NO," when I asked if Lindsey could go to early childhood classes in both the morning and afternoon sessions. Everyone agreed that the early childhood classes were helping her, yet the director of special education said, "If we do this for her, all moms will want us to do this for their children." I felt like they thought I was trying to get rid of my child for the day. That was not my intention. I wanted her to have more help, and all of the research along with Lyle Chastain's recommendations pointed in that direction.

Discouraged, I left the meeting in tears and went home to talk to Todd. When Todd walked in the door from work, I said, "Let's move. I am not going to spend all of Lindsey's school years fighting for help."

Todd was beyond supportive and told me to start looking for what I thought would be a better situation for our family. The following day, I started calling the surrounding school districts. My best response came from the early childhood teachers in a town about 20 miles away. We set up a visit with them the very next day. They even told me that I should bring Lindsey with me.

Lindsey, not liking new situations, behaved exactly how I expected she would. I could barely get her to walk through the doorway and into the room. As soon as she entered the room, she walked over to a shelf full of toys and books, and using her arm, she swiped the shelf clean. One of the early childhood teachers and the speech therapist were present for the whole thing. Neither of them had a big reaction as Lindsey continued to cry, scream, and tried to play with the toys. I don't remember much else from the meeting, but I do remember their final words.

The early childhood teacher said, "We are up for the challenge. Lindsey can attend both the morning and afternoon sessions." They informed me that the afternoon session would be a repeat of the morning session. I couldn't believe what I was hearing especially after what they had just witnessed.

On the drive home, I was so excited to tell Todd. Todd immediately searched for a lot in town to build our new home. It didn't matter to him that it would extend his commute to work; he wanted us to be happy. I was grateful. Lindsey continued to go to her current school until we moved.

Chapter Twenty-Four

"Grandma with the Camera"

By Ida Feyereisen, Lindsey's Grandma

Lindsey was a beautiful little girl with light brown hair and big blue eyes, but she had a hard time making eye contact. When she was very young, I learned that I could put a camera between her face and mine, and apparently the curiosity of the object in front of me, held her attention long enough for me to get a picture of her. It also allowed me to look into her eyes for just that split second. Not all picture-taking attempts were successful. I, like most people my age, don't have a lot of pictures of my childhood or even of my own children. Maybe that's the reason I like to take pictures of my fifteen grandchildren. I may be remembered as "The Grandma with the Camera," but someday I hope they look back at the memories and enjoy my pictures and the picture taking experiences. Lindsey wasn't comfortable being close to other people, so for that reason group pictures were hard for her.

As proud grandparents, we started sending out picture Christmas cards when the grandchildren were young. I tried to come up with a unique idea each year. In 1997, I got the idea to do a live nativity scene. At that point, we had twelve grandchildren ranging in age from 4 months to 8 years. I was excited and even spent hours sewing the costumes. We had Baby Jesus, Mary, Joseph, a shepherd, a Wiseman, a cow, a sheep, two angels, a donkey, a cat (doesn't every stable need one?), and a very special star. At 3 years and 11 months, Lindsey was still having a problem with the sensation of clothes touching her skin. She didn't like anything on her body, but tolerated some t-shirts. So, I decided to sew a star to the front of one of Lindsey's comfortable t-shirts. But in case that didn't interest her, I had a backup plan and made her a cardboard star on the end of a paint stick that I hoped she would hold up over the group of people and animals in the stable. In the days and weeks leading up to the scheduled Thanksgiving Day picture-taking-event, we kept showing her the shirt and the star on the stick. We kept telling her she was going to be the special star of Bethlehem. We could only hope that she would cooperate, but I'm sure I wasn't the only one who had my doubts. They arrived at our house early that day and much to our surprise she wanted to put the shirt on, and even more of a surprise was the fact that she also wanted to hold the star on the stick. For her, it wasn't one or the other. She wanted both. This was the moment I realized that Lindsey really wanted to socialize, but it didn't take me long to figure out that even though it might be what she wanted, it wasn't going to be easy for her. Brittany was now dressed as Mary, and soon the other actors began to arrive. By the time they were all dressed and in position, Lindsey could not bring herself to join the group. Since she now seemed happy to both wear the t-shirt and hold the star, we positioned a stool for her to sit on behind the other kids. We hoped she would sit there and hold up the star. But, you've guessed it again. She wanted nothing to do with this whole nativity scene business. Obviously, this was just a proud grandma's dream to show off the grandkids. I'm sure only a few of the kids were old enough at the time to understand the Christmas story.

After putting Lauri, Todd, Brittany and the whole cast of characters, along with their parents, through a lot of stress, we got our picture. Lauri would sit Lindsey on the stool and give her a kernel of popcorn, which was her one food cravings at the time. We had about two seconds to snap a picture, and she was gone. Baby Jesus kept slipping out of the well-padded wicker clothes basket, the cow kept crawling off the platform, and the sheep was shedding tears after being awakened from a nap. All parents kept repositioning their kids after each shot, and Lauri kept returning Lindsey to the stool and handing her another piece of popcorn. This was long before the use of digital cameras (at least in our family) so of course I wanted several shots to make sure we would get one good one. My sister Pat took many pictures and ran them into Wal-Mart's one-hour photo so we could pick one that day and get the Christmas cards printed and in the mail in time for Christmas. In the end, I guess Lindsey knew best when she insisted on holding the star pointing down. Since our room was small and the photographers couldn't get back any farther, it was the only way the "Star" (who was wearing the star t-shirt, and holding the star on the stick) were all in the picture with the other actors. The cards were great and family and friends enjoyed them. We've been told this was a favorite.

Chapter Twenty-Five

"I need help"

By Ida Feyereisen, Lindsey's Grandma

At our house, when she was able to play alone without any of the other grandchildren around, Lindsey played quietly by herself in our basement toy room. Most of the time, to my surprise, she played at the little white dish cupboard that my dad had made when I was 4 years old. She played with the plastic dishes and the fake food. It was surprising to me that she liked putting two pieces of plastic bread together with realistic looking plastic sandwich fillings like tomatoes, lettuce, hamburger, pickles, and even butter. There was no way Lindsey would eat a sandwich like this, with her self-imposed diet, but she took delight in serving it to me on a little plastic plate. I always told her how good it was, and pretended to eat every bite. I always clearly named each ingredient in the hopes that someday she would repeat just one word.

One day when Lindsey was about 4 or 4-1/2, Lauri and I sat at the kitchen table visiting while Lindsey quietly played in the basement. My heart skipped a beat, and my stomach rose to my lungs, leaving the feeling that I wouldn't get my next breath. I had just heard the most spectacular three little words that I had ever heard come from the playroom in our basement. "I need help!"

Lindsey had spoken her first sentence, and could it really be that changes for the good were truly here to stay? Could this mean the silent world of frustration for her and her family would now be in the past? Her mother and I rushed to the basement as if the house was on fire.

Lindsey was sitting on the toilet, and yes she needed help. These were not her first words, but for the first time in all these hard, frustrating days and nights for 4 ½ long years, Lindsey had spoken a sentence, and not just any sentence, she had asked for help. She had identified herself, and shown a need for others. Could it really last?

Chapter Twenty-Six

"Speech therapy to the rescue!"

By Lauri Moreland, Lindsey's mom

During the process of writing this book and reflecting on Lindsey's progress, I came across home videos of Lindsey on VHS. We don't have a VHS player anymore, so I had them converted to DVDs. I watched the video of the day Lindsey was diagnosed with autism. It is stuck in my head and my heart. I had forgotten how severe her tantrums were and how she was unable to communicate with us in a respectful manner. Imagine a 28 month old toddler screaming as she climbed up a bar stool, onto a counter, batting at objects, and impatiently waiting for what she wanted. The problem was we didn't know what she wanted. The image can be compared to a baby anxiously awaiting a bottle at the perfect temperature and perfect angle. However, with a baby there is only one choice, that bottle. With Lindsey, we did our best to guess. On this day, I guessed toast with syrup on it. The toast had to be the correct color with the exact amount of syrup she liked or the screaming would never end. To top that, it had to be cut in little squares, approximately nine bites. Still, it was not fast enough for Lindsey.

Thinking about this, I realized that by the time we moved to the new school district, she had already made some improvements. At 4 ½ years, Lindsey spoke that first sentence. As my mom put it well, it wasn't just a sentence, it was a sentence in which she was advocating for herself appropriately.

Lindsey went to preschool all day, five days a week. The afternoon session was a repeat of the morning which proved to benefit her. There were good days and bad days, yet I knew it was exactly where she needed to be each day. Speech therapy at school was part of her IEP. In addition, she had occupational therapy. Although she responded well to all of the teachers, she was especially fond of her classroom teacher and her speech therapist. They were our super heroes when it came to helping Lindsey communicate with us. Even though we had already been using the Mayer Johnson Symbols and sign language, we were all ready for the next challenge…speaking.

Her teachers were patient, gentle, accommodating, and Lindsey's biggest cheerleaders. They had an instant connection with her. We kept a communication notebook so that we could reinforce everything that was working well at school along with using the same language. We identified what Lindsey was doing verbally to her such as, "Lindsey is walking, Lindsey is jumping, and Lindsey is eating." We also identified her emotions for her such as, "Lindsey is happy or Lindsey is sad."

We all felt that we had the support system of the entire school district backing us up. Because Lindsey was one of the first children to have an autism diagnosis in the district, the entire staff was eager to learn more about autism and more importantly how to help Lindsey. Her speech therapist continued to work with her through third grade. She had wonderful teachers each year. They implemented a friendship group, a cooking class to help with her limited diet, and provided her a safe resource room to go to when she needed sensory therapy or a place to work through unexpected behaviors.

Lindsey loved all of her teachers so much. In kindergarten, the school district sent both her kindergarten teacher and me to a conference to learn more about autism. It was a week-long conference and her teacher and I learned a lot about how to be partners in Lindsey's education. The parent/teacher partnership proved to be essential in the advancement of her academic and social growth. As Lindsey's language progressed, she was able to tell us how much she truly loved her teachers.

The progress Lindsey was making in elementary school was enormous. Yet, there were daily challenges and tantrums. When I look at Lindsey now and I have conversations with her, I question, "Was it really that bad? Did her autism present itself in such significant ways?" The videos are a reminder that it was. At the time, it felt strange to videotape our little girl behaving in a way that not only puzzled me, but also made me wonder what her future would be like without being able to communicate effectively. I am grateful for the videos even though they are hard to watch. Lindsey leaves the room when we watch them. She is glad she doesn't remember these moments.

It was about this time that we were hit with another blow. We had seen Brittany's face and fingers shake on different occasions. I had taken her to the doctor 3 times and was assured each time that it was just a nervous twitch. I was working one Saturday morning and Brittany was visiting her cousin Kayla and Aunt Linda when she had her first grand mal seizure. That was the start of Brittany's life with epilepsy.

I thought autism was the worst thing in the world, but there were many times that Brittany's struggles with epilepsy were even worse.

Chapter Twenty-Seven

"My teachers were my friends."

By Lindsey Moreland

The early childhood teachers were taking a class picture. I was probably four years old. I wanted no part of that. I hid under the desk whining and letting people know that I didn't want to be by others. I wanted to be alone and standing next to others for what seemed to be no sensible reason wasn't what I wanted to do. I needed my space and came out from under the table only after the teachers said the pictures were all done. I hid under the table because I didn't like it when people looked at me. Now, they were even asking me to smile. It was confusing and scary. I couldn't communicate my thinking like the other kids.

Skip ahead to kindergarten. I loved my teacher. She was my favorite. She was sweet, kind, and supportive. She understood me and didn't pretend to like me like some other people do. I felt like she liked me regardless of what I could do and what I couldn't do. She was always there for me. When our class went on a field trip to another school to watch the play *The Jungle Book,* I remember getting scared when we got to meet the characters after the play. I was scared of the character *Shere Kahn,* the evil tiger. I couldn't figure out why no one else was scared. I didn't realize that it was just a guy dressed up and playing the part. I freaked out. He wanted to shake my hand, and I couldn't do it. My teacher hugged me tight and calmed me down. She didn't care that the other students weren't scared. She just wanted to help me.

Figuring out what was right and wrong was confusing for me. One time in kindergarten, I started kicking classmates on the playground. It was a sunny day, and for some reason I felt like kicking. Of course, the classmates told on me and I got in trouble. My teacher was disappointed in me and walked me to the special education room. The special education teacher talked to me about it and had me apologize to the classmate. I was accepted back into the classroom and treated well because I had made it all better. I learned my lesson.

In first grade, I wanted a birthday party. My mom asked, "Who would you like to invite to your birthday party?" I responded, "My friends." When my mom asked me to name my friends, I named my kindergarten teacher, my first grade teacher, my special education teacher, my speech teacher, my aide and her son, who was in my class. My mom tried to explain that teachers don't typically come to a student's birthday party, but I insisted that we ask. My teachers were my friends. I wanted my family, too, but my friends were my teachers and I wanted them there. To my mom's surprise, every single one of my teachers came. My mom was overjoyed by the support.

I always seemed to say what I was thinking at this age. My speech was broken, but apparently my speech teacher was doing a good job because I was beginning to talk a lot. I announced to the whole birthday party that my Aunt Nancy had lost her front tooth. I don't remember announcing this, but my mom reminded me of it. Aunt Nancy didn't want to come to the party because of some dental issues she had at the time. I was proud she had lost a tooth because I was at the age when the tooth fairy paid me for my lost teeth. My mom says this was the turning point in my language development. I was beginning to try out more words and put sentences together. For example, I tried saying, "I am six years old." It came out, "I am sick year old." Whatever the words, I wanted to talk, but sometimes my talking was uncomfortable for my family and those around me.

Not all teachers understood me. I specifically remember a second grade spelling test. I had gotten one wrong and all of the other words correct. The word was neighbors. I spelled it "n-i-e-g-h-b-o-r-s" mixing up the vowel pattern. Wasn't the rule "i before e-except after c"?

"How come this world can't follow rules?" I wondered. I argued with my teacher, and today I admit that my attitude was bad. She sent me in the hallway, and I sat on the floor. I was angry. Years passed, and I shared the experience with my mom. I wished I would have had the words to explain how I was feeling. As an adult, I can see the humor in my thinking, but at the time I felt upset and embarrassed to be put in the hallway.

I was content with my teachers being my friends, and I wanted to please them. That is not what my teachers wanted for me, though. My teachers wanted me to have friends my own age. I didn't understand why at the time. Plus, I didn't like the lunch room. I didn't like the playground. The lunch room was noisy and there were lots of people. I preferred to eat lunch in the special education classroom where it was quiet. On the playground, I wanted to play alone. The teachers wanted me to interact with other classmates. I felt like I had more freedom when I could play by myself. "If you don't go to lunch or to the playground, it's going to be hard to make friends," my teachers said.

Yet, the lunchroom and the playground were unpredictable. Every day it was different. Would the swings be full or would someone already be in my favorite swing? Would other kids get too close to me when I was standing in line to get on the slide? Would the playground teacher make me play a game with other students, or could I be left alone that day? Would the person sitting by me at lunch have smelly food, and I would need to plug my nose? There were just too many things I couldn't predict. I liked eating my two s'more Pop Tarts, my grapes, my Cheetos, and my milk with no one to bother me.

Some people reading this might wonder, "Is this a spoiled little girl just trying to get what she wants?" My mother said that my great grandmother (who I share a birthday with) once said that I just needed a good old fashioned spanking. That's not how autism works. When things change and don't go the way they are planned, my body reacts in certain ways. When I was younger, I screamed and threw myself to the ground. I would bang my head on concrete and sometimes my whole body. The words weren't there for me like other children. As an adult, I get a headache and stomach aches. I sometimes have to pace back and forth to calm myself down. I don't like admitting this, but I have a nervous habit of picking my fingernails when I have anxiety. It takes time to get over it. It helps me to go off by myself and just be by myself until it goes away.

Chapter Twenty-Eight

"What is the meaning of friendship?"

By Lauri Moreland, Lindsey's mom

Elementary school to me was a time to make friends and play with classmates. I was a shy little girl and a bit unsure of myself, yet I had the courage to approach my classmates when it came time to choose a partner or join a game on the playground. I always had someone to sit with on the bus, and I always had someone to sit by during lunch. My sister reminds me that when her friends came to our house, I always joined in whether she wanted me to or not. As an adult, I have no shortage of friends, and I love being social. I have been told that I am one of the first to arrive and the last to leave a gathering.

I imagined that my own children would be similar to me and have no trouble making friends or keeping friends. No one ever had to teach me what to do to make a friend. It seemed to be a natural part of growing up. Thinking of my teachers as my friends would be the last thing on my mind. I didn't spend my time thinking about homework or the grade I would get on an assignment. I was thinking of hanging out with others my own age.

My heart hurt that Lindsey didn't have friends her age. It made me happy that she liked her teachers well enough to consider them friends. I give them tons of credit, and it says a lot about the important role they played in her growing up years. We all just assumed that Lindsey wanted to spend time with others her own age, but that was just confusing for her. She expressed interest in being invited to birthday parties, and she wanted classmates to come play at her house.

Her teachers and I became her friendship coordinators doing our best to try to include her in any way possible. When Lindsey did invite someone over, the play time stamina for her was short. Within half an hour, she was done playing with them and wanted to be left alone. Brittany would end up playing with the guest. Lindsey liked the idea of having a friend, and I hoped that someday she would experience the true meaning of friendship. To me, the true meaning of friendship is a give and take equal relationship with another person that is built on trust and understanding. This was all foreign to her.

What can we do to help not only children with autism, but all children feel wanted and accepted? What can we do to ensure that children have true friends? I wondered and worried about this. I know that teachers and parents can't "make" friendships happen. Lindsey's elementary school had many supports in place to help her. She got to invite classmates to eat with her in a quiet area, play with her in a resource room, and enjoy occupational therapy toys with her. I was grateful, but also sad at the same time. I didn't want her to need these supports. In elementary school, most classmates were eager to be involved in Lindsey's day. Unfortunately, it didn't result in invitations from them or lasting friendships. In fact, in all of her school years, she was only invited to two different parties, both were in elementary school.

When it was time for Lindsey to move on to middle school, I was hopeful that this would be her time to learn how to make a friend and be a friend. Middle school started in 5th grade. She continued to get a great amount of academic support through special education and social skills instruction. As her classmates became middle schoolers, they became more independent while their friendships grew and changed along the way. Could I say they were mean to her? Yes and No. In my opinion, maybe some of them didn't understand and they went about their day oblivious to her existence. When they did notice her, she was the strange kid, the weird kid, and mostly the kid that wouldn't look at other students. Why couldn't they have tried harder to include her? I recognize that middle school is hard enough as adolescents are trying to make sense of the world and are trying to fit in with others. I was mad inside that at least one student wouldn't step up and try to be her friend. I wished I had been that one student in middle school who would have stepped up to be a friend to a child with special needs. I was not that kid. I had friends, but I also had insecurities. I was overweight and struggled academically.

Upon talking to a few of Lindsey's classmates after high school graduation, they were shocked that she felt left out. At that point, I had a hard time believing them. They told my nephew they truly thought she preferred to be left alone. Educating the students about autism may have made a difference...but maybe not.

Twenty-two years ago, I was told by a therapist that 1 in 10,000 kids were being diagnosed with autism. I'm seeing different numbers, but as of today, most sources are saying it's 1 in 68.

Summers were hell. Lindsey needed a schedule. It was hard to fill her day. This would have been a good time to have more therapy. There really wasn't anything available. At this point, she didn't need OT, PT, or speech. I do feel that she would have benefited from more sensory therapy at a center. The days and early evenings felt like forever. She wandered around the house looking lost. We did what we could. We are very lucky that our friend Judith, who was a mentor to the girls, had a horse farm. My schedule was not always great to be able to get them to her farm. Sometimes, she came to pick them up. She never took any money from us. She gave the girls riding lessons. The girls were always welcome to ride. Both girls benefited from their time with Judith. She was always patient and kind.

I had gone to cosmetology school right out of high school and had worked part time until we moved to Iowa. About 9 months after we moved back to Wisconsin I started working 3 evenings a week and Todd had the girls. By the time the girls were in middle school I was working almost full time. I made time in my busy schedule to take the girls to the community pool, and I played a lot of cards and board games with Lindsey. We watched movies together, and we baked gluten free treats. Her classmates were busy with their friends. Unfortunately, she was not included.

What does a mother do next? Hire a friend. Yes, you read that right. We hired a friend for Lindsey. Margaret was a sweet girl that was also a client of mine that I cut hair for. She was in high school and was looking for a summer job. I paid her to come one day a week to hang out with Lindsey. At the time, we didn't tell Lindsey that we were employing someone to be her friend. She loved her time with her "friend" Margaret. They went for walks to a nearby lake, they played in a tree house outside, played cards, and played board games. Margaret learned quickly that each activity was short, sweet, and to the point when it came to being Lindsey's friend. Although I was grateful for Margaret and got used to paying her each week, I still couldn't believe I had to hire someone to hang out with my middle school daughter. Throughout the years, I met many parents and enjoyed hearing about their children and their social activities with other children their age, but I couldn't shake the fact that we were replacing real childhood friendships with a hired "friend." People often told me, "Lindsey is doing great for having autism," but hiring Margaret to interact with Lindsey was a daily reminder of how different our life was compared to other families. It was hard to feel like it was fair. A mother doesn't want to have these feelings, but they can't be ignored. It was a constant tug on my heart. Would Lindsey ever understand or experience my true meaning of friendship?

Chapter Twenty-Nine

"Same Matters"

By Ida Feyereisen, Lindsey's grandma

The following is a page from my journal when Lindsey was 11, and in 3rd or 4th grade:

Food always was, and may always be a problem for Lindsey. For some reason that the rest of us don't understand, she just can't bring herself to eat most food items we all eat without batting an eye. We know sometimes it's the smell, but perhaps it's the texture, or the taste that could lead her to starvation rather than even try something new. Eating at home was problem enough, but eating at school, or at our house or anyone else's house was way worse. Burger King's chicken nuggets were an accepted food item for many years, and believe me, Lauri & Todd bought a lot of them. Attempts to put other nuggets in Burger King Wrappers always failed. She knew better, and she would not eat them.

The elementary school system and the special education teachers were great! I can't stress that enough. They knew Lindsey had a hard time with food. In about 3rd or 4th grade they created a way to introduce new food into her diet with hopes of expanding her limited self-imposed diet. Lindsey was allowed to pick two other classmates to come to cooking class with her. They chose menus, prepared, and ATE the food. I believe they had to at least try everything. When they were working on a unit in class honoring Dr. Seuss, they made green eggs and ham. Much to our surprise Lindsey ate this and wanted it at home. For months, Lauri made "Green Eggs and Ham" every day, but then one day Lindsey was "all done" or at least said "not today."

These were two phrases we have heard a lot since she first started to talk at age four. Once I got real excited when I heard that Lindsey was eating canned, whole kernel corn. I went out and bought a few cans of the **exact brand** to have on hand, and Lindsey would eat the whole can-nothing with it, just the corn. Then one day, when they came to our house, I was out of the canned corn, so I went to the freezer and got out some of our good homegrown frozen corn. Lindsey was outside playing when I cooked it. I was sure she wouldn't be able to tell the difference, but you guessed it, she could tell. Now she didn't trust corn at our house ever again. Even if I show her the can she just says, "Not today." In fact, she really doesn't trust anything I try to cook for her. It's a lot easier if she just packs her lunch and eats it by herself before the rest of the family is served. It hurts me to see her have to do this, and I want so badly for her to someday let me cook something new and special just for her, and have her eat it. I don't ever remember her saying "no" or that she didn't like something at my house. She always uses those phrases like "not today," "all done," or in later years, "same matters"-as in the same can of corn, the same brand of chips, and the same kind of bread and the same pans. Yes, they even brought their "same" pans to our house to make her green eggs & ham.

When I wrote that story in my journal so many years ago, I would never have dreamed I would live to see Lindsey sitting at our table with a plate of food in front of her and her cousins around her. Today, as an adult, Lindsey is a great eater. She eats everything: meat, fruits, vegetables, salads, and gluten free desserts.

Chapter Thirty
"Gluten-free pays off!"
By Lauri Moreland

I was diagnosed with celiac disease in 2002. I had stomach aches all of my life which was not only extremely painful, but also led to multiple hospital stays. At one point, I thought I would have to quit my job because of how sick I was. When my family doctor ran a blood test and it came back positive, I knew my life would change. A biopsy would confirm the diagnosis. I was instructed to strictly follow a gluten free diet. I learned that even a cross contamination of food could send me to the hospital.

After I was diagnosed, I questioned if Lindsey also had celiac disease. Lindsey had stomach issues from birth. She vomited often. Unfortunately, she couldn't tell us that she was hurting. She would wake up in the middle of the night and vomit. There were times when she would be so ill that she would tear the lining in her stomach. This would result in hospitalization which would typically last for about two days. We decided to have Lindsey tested for celiac disease. Her blood test came back positive which led to a biopsy. Her biopsy came back negative. We were confused, yet relieved and happy she didn't have it. We told her that she could eat whatever she wanted. To our dismay, she continued to get ill and vomited often. Our doctor explained that there are times that a biopsy can be a false read or be inconclusive. Our doctor felt strongly that Lindsey indeed did have celiac disease and needed her to start eating gluten free. Desperate for answers and change, I sat down with Lindsey and had a conversation with her about her diet.

I wanted her to try the gluten free diet to see if it would help her feel better. With the limited amount of things she was willing to eat, I was worried about how she would survive eating just gluten free food. She was small framed and already underweight. Because Lindsey was tired of throwing up, tired of doctor visits, and tired of needing IV fluids for dehydration, she was willing to try it. I was grateful that she understood the importance of trying it. I knew that if we had tried it earlier in her life when she couldn't communicate with us at all, she would have starved herself to death.

Week one of the diet, I noticed a tremendous change in her behavior. I had never seen her so calm. The throwing up ceased. Weeks on the diet turned into months and years. It was the end of the hospital stays. With my experience on the diet and experimenting with some terrible tasting foods and some great tasting foods, I was able to introduce her to gluten free foods that she would actually eat. I was cooking and baking with flours and ingredients that I never knew existed before I had been diagnosed. Once I discovered them, I also became aware of the astronomical cost of going gluten free. None of that mattered to me if Lindsey was going to feel better and behave better.

Although Todd and Brittany did not need to be on this special diet, they were willing to try foods with us. Todd would even pick up foods he would see at the store that were gluten free. He would be excited when he found a new item that we might try. Todd and Brittany still eat foods with gluten in them but are careful to make sure that they don't cross contaminate their food with ours.

In my opinion, going gluten free resulted in the biggest, most positive change for Lindsey. Not only was she calmer and better behaved, she had the patience to try and communicate with us using her words. When she got frustrated, she didn't throw a major temper tantrum. She wasn't hitting herself as much anymore, either. In conclusion, for Lindsey, going gluten free paid off for all of us.

Chapter Thirty-One

"Talking about my passions helps me be more social."

By Lindsey Moreland

I have memories of growing up that I can look back on now and chuckle or smile. When you read them, you will get a glimpse of what an autistic child's brain might be thinking, or at least what my brain was thinking, growing up.

When I was young, I always wanted a pet fish because I thought it would be easy to take care of for me. I loved the movie *Finding Nemo*, so I wanted a Pacific Blue Tang just like Dory in the movie. I wanted to name it Mae because I thought it was pretty unique. To prepare for getting the fish and to convince my mom that I could handle a fish, I found a shoebox at home in the storage room. After writing the name Mae on the top, I brought it to my mom.

She asked, "What is the shoebox for?"

I replied, "I know animals die, so I have a coffin prepared for Mae when she dies."

My mom tried not to laugh and reminded me that I didn't even have a fish. You may wonder if I ever got the fish. Sadly, I did not. I kept the shoebox for a while and decided to store other treasures in it.

When I was 8 ½ years old, I was listening to a live album of Elvis Presley, and I asked my family, "Who is that singing?"

My dad told me, "That's Elvis Presley." He told me that he was a great singer and also said he died in 1977.

I couldn't stop listening to Elvis Presley. I listened in the morning before school and after. I checked out books about him and began memorizing facts:

Elvis Aron Presley

Born-January 8, 1935

Death-August 16, 1977

Married to Priscilla-May 1, 1967

I could go on and on about Elvis. Thankfully, I was encouraged to learn more about him because it helped me learn, and it also gave me something to talk about with other people. I could impress them with my knowledge. I felt happy when people asked me about what I knew. I am still interested in Elvis, but learning about Elvis also led me to other passions.

At age 11, my family and I went to Orlando, Florida for a vacation. We went to Sea World, Universal Studios, Magic Kingdom and Animal Kingdom at Disney World, Pirates' Dinner Show, and the Titanic Exhibit Museum.

"What is Titanic?" I wondered. I had never heard of it before. After learning about the history of the greatest ocean liner, I became fascinated with it. Becoming fascinated or obsessed with a special interest is typical of many people with autism. I am grateful that my family has always let me pursue my special interests.

My favorite part of the museum was when my sister and I were the only ones who got the opportunity to walk up and down the first class grand staircase because the grand staircase is one of my favorite rooms from the Titanic. Employees handed us passenger tickets. My passenger ticket was Jean Gertrude Hippach, a 16 year old from first class. Brittany's ticket was Michel Navratil, second class passenger. He was an orphan whose father kidnapped him with his younger brother after his father lost custody of his boys. I don't remember who Mom was, but Dad's ticket was Margaret "Molly" Brown, the well-known first class passenger. The details about the passengers, the construction of the ship, the maiden voyage, and the sinking furthered my curiosity and fascination with Titanic.

When I was 12 years old, I watched the James Cameron 1997 film, *Titanic*. I thought it was a true story because it was based on the history of the sinking Titanic. However, I didn't realize that it was a historical film and the characters were just acting the part. It was confusing for me because some of the characters' story lines were fiction while others were real. After watching it, I was in tears because of Leonardo DiCaprio's character's death. He became my first celebrity crush, and still is today!

I thought that poor Leonardo DiCaprio actually died, and they filmed his death. How awful. It was devastating for me. Looking back on it now, I realize how silly it was, yet one day I printed a picture of Jack Dawson (Leonardo's character), and I wrote a grave saying, "In Loving Memory of Jack Dawson, 1890-1912." I put it on top of my curio shelf in my bedroom. Again, my family chuckled at the very quirky me.

My love for the Titanic did not end here. I began drawing the ship, almost every single day. In seventh and eighth grade, I drew it before the sinking and after the sinking. I couldn't think of anything else, except the Titanic. Every time I went to the library, I would rather check out books on it than any other books there. I even designed the cover for my assignment notebook with the theme being the Titanic. Using pictures I had printed off from both the film and history, I added the words, "I Love Titanic." I completed it with hearts drawn around each picture. That same year, someone saw my notebook and wrote, "I love Titanic, too, Lindsey!" on it. I was curious who wrote it. I felt appreciated for my love of my interest. I never found out who did it, and I have always wondered who it was. You might wonder why all of these details are important.

During high school, I painted a couple canvases of Titanic, and even one of it sinking. In the summer of 2009, my aunt Linda took me to the Science Museum in St. Paul, Minnesota to see the Titanic Exhibit and watch the IMAX movie of the Titanic wreck. Just like Florida, we had passenger tickets. Mine was from second class. My aunt was lucky because her passenger ticket was from first class. Our passengers did survive the sinking, thank goodness. In my opinion, being able to have these experiences is important. I hope that other families who have children with autism will encourage them to follow their passions and obsessions in a positive way.

Furthering my interest, in 2012, the 100th year anniversary of the Titanic, Brittany, Mom, and I saw *Titanic* in 3-D. It was the greatest Easter gift from Mom because it was really cool seeing my favorite film in the theater. It is great that we can continue to learn. In my first year of technical college I was in a writing class, and I learned a new fact about the James Cameron 1997 film. Since Jack Dawson was from Wisconsin, he told Rose that he used to go fishing at Lake Wissota while convincing her not to jump off the Titanic. The history of the Titanic happened in 1912, but Lake Wissota didn't exist until 1918. I don't know what James Cameron was thinking, but it was sure a fine idea to add on his screenplay! My thinking when I learned this was that the fact was interesting and seemed unlikely, yet I was and am glad that this film received 11 Oscars, including Best Picture.

Since I have been fascinated with Titanic, I have been collecting books, magazines, posters, artwork, childhood artwork, entertainment, puzzles, memorabilia, and so much more. I hope to have a replica of the ship model someday. I also designed my website of my Titanic collection: http://lindseymoreland.wix.com/titanic. My dream will be complete with a visit to Branson, Missouri to see America's largest Titanic museum attraction. I would love to travel to Belfast in Northern Ireland to see the museum, at the exact spot where Titanic was constructed in the 1900's and was launched on May 31, 1911. I would also love to travel to Southampton, England to see the dock where Titanic started her maiden voyage on April 10, 1912.

Again, I am grateful my family lets me explore my interest. I truly believe I have become a better reader and a better artist. I am able to memorize many facts when I am interested in the subject. Being able to talk about things that interest me, helps me be more social. I like it when people ask me about my passions. It makes me feel included in conversations. It also makes it easier for me to talk to other people when I am confident about what I have to say.

Chapter Thirty-Two

"Lindsey was in a play."

By Ida Feyereisen, Lindsey's grandma

Our lower level family room isn't used regularly anymore now that our children are all grown, and even the grandchildren have become young adults. On holidays and special occasions, it thrills me to no end to see it packed with our growing family. One day I walked into that room and looked at the huge bookcase full of photo albums. It reminded me that Lindsey was the one who enjoyed the pictures the most. Starting at a very young age, even before she talked, Lindsey would spend hours at a time quietly looking through those albums as the rest of the family sat at the kitchen table visiting or playing cards.

On this particular day, I randomly pulled out the one marked 2005 and slowly turned the pages filled with many wonderful memories of the kids and grandkids. I found Lindsey on her birthday, her sister Brittany's birthday, and several cousins' birthday parties. There she was with the group of cousins. As the year went on, she seemed to be mixing more with the group and not always staying on the far left or right. As I looked through the pictures, I enjoyed remembering the grandkids playing football, baseball, and softball. There were pictures of piano recitals, band &

choir concerts, dancers, runners, gymnasts, horseback riders, and actors in plays and musicals. "Wait!" I said to myself. "Why wasn't there a picture of Lindsey in her first school play? This should be the year for that." For a while I couldn't remember the play or the part she played. As the years go by, I'm so glad I have these pictures to help jar my aging memory, and of course there is always the option to call the kids.

I called Lauri, and she asked Lindsey about her school play. She quickly replied that her first school play was in 2005. Why then, I asked Lauri don't I have any pictures of that? She said that I was videotaping it that year, and they had the video. I still felt very bad that I didn't have any pictures in the photo album of Lindsey in her first play. I started to close that old album with the pictures falling out. There it was. How could I have missed it? It was a very special picture of the most beautiful eleven year old girl dressed in her Native American girl outfit. Her mother and sister were in it also, and Lindsey had a huge smile on her face, holding an arm full of flowers. Now I remembered! The play was Lewis and Clark, and Lindsey had talked about it for weeks. Her class had studied the Lewis and Clark expedition. She had told me all about it and about the Native Americans they had met along their way. She would be a Native American in the play. She was so excited.

I was excited too and so proud that she was going to actually act in a school play. She had come so far, but there was no denying there were still many social issues. In the days leading up to the big day, I was nervous. I was worried for her. Would she run off the stage and not go through with it? Would she forget where to stand and what to do? Would the other kids make fun of her or tease her about something? She wasn't worried, nervous, or afraid, so why on earth should I have been? She was great! I couldn't have been more proud. There would be wonderful things ahead for her. I just knew it! There was no stopping her now.

Chapter Thirty-Three

"Took the magazine and covered my face."

By Lindsey Moreland

Growing up with autism was my secret. I didn't want others to know because I thought maybe they would think that I was a bad person. I didn't want them to think or say something bad about me. Saying the word autism felt like it was a bad thing. I don't think that way now, but at the time I did. I just wanted to be looked at as "normal" like everyone else. When I am embarrassed, I want whatever I am embarrassed about to be a secret.

Not only having autism was a secret for me growing up, but also being involved in a very serious accident. I rarely talk about it. In the summer of 2005, I joined the girls' softball team for middle school. When I was younger, I enjoyed playing t-ball, so I thought I would also enjoy softball. I wanted to be a part of a team or group. I thought it would help me make friends and fit in with the other girls.

I was 11 years old and I just finished 5th grade. I liked playing softball with the girls and felt like I was doing well socializing and hanging out with them. We had been losing all of our games, except for one, but it was worth it to me to have fun. My favorite position was pitching. I remembered that I was good at it.

The day my accident happened, it was a sunny July day. Mom and I went to the game in a small town in Wisconsin. The coach told me that in the second half I was going to get to be the pitcher. I was so excited. In the first half, I was playing second base, but I couldn't wait to play pitcher. The girls on the other team were taller and bigger than most of the girls on our team. It seemed like they were probably 8th graders going into high school in the fall.

It was the middle of the game, and I still hadn't got my chance to pitch. I was playing second base when a tall girl from the opposite team got up to bat. She hit a line drive towards me. I was paying close attention and thought I was ready to catch the ball. The softball hit my cheek, and I screamed as I fell to the sand. All of my team members came over to me immediately, but I couldn't handle being around too many people at that moment. My mom and some of the other parents came over and my mom mentioned that I needed more space. As I was lying down, one of the ladies who happened to be a doctor told me that I needed to sit up, otherwise it would get worse.

I was scared and puzzled. I could feel my cheek swelling. My mom wanted to drive me to the hospital in our home town to see my own doctor, but was told that it was too far of a drive. I needed medical attention immediately, and I needed to go to the local hospital. As my mom and I were driving to the emergency room, it was getting worse. At the emergency room, my mom called my sister Brittany to let her know what happened to me. Brittany felt bad because it was the only game she had missed. I also remember my mom trying to get ahold of my dad at work, but she couldn't reach him because no one was in the office to answer the phones at night.

I was watching the clock as the minutes ticked by, and we were in the emergency room for nearly four hours. I was scared for many reasons. I was in pain and I was worried that the nurse was going to stick an IV needle in me. I have an extreme fear of needles, but thank goodness there were no needles!

When the doctor came in and told me that my cheekbone was broken, I was scared. He said that I was lucky because if the softball hit at a different spot other than my cheek, it could have been much more serious. My mom wanted to take a picture of my face, but after seeing myself in front of the mirror, I refused to let her take the picture. I felt ugly... Only one picture was eventually taken.

When I got home from the hospital, my sister started crying because she saw my face. Not only was my face very swollen, it also looked like the laces from the ball were planted in my face. I tried to comfort her and tell her that it was going to be ok. I felt dirty from the softball game and went to take a bath. My sister stayed by my side as my mom helped scrub my body carefully. Afterward, I had some ice cream to make me feel better. Instead of lying down on my bed, I had to sit up and sleep which was uncomfortable. I had to sit up while sleeping so the blood flow wouldn't get worse. It was difficult to sleep because my face still felt swollen. When my dad got home from work, I heard my mom say, "Go up to the loft and look at Lindsey." Because I was having a hard time sleeping, my eyes kept on opening and closing. I saw my dad looking shocked when he saw my face. I was comforted that my parents and sister cared so much for me.

The next day, I had a doctor's appointment somewhere in Minnesota. We had to ride an elevator to get the doctor's office. People were staring at me and I could feel their stares. I did not like that at all, and I was embarrassed. I put my hands over my face because I didn't want anyone seeing me or making comments about me. In the waiting room, more people were staring at me, so I took the magazine that was nearby and covered my face. My mom protected my feelings by telling the people that were staring that I broke cheekbone in a softball accident. After my mom shared the story, people understood and respected my privacy.

A couple days later after the accident, I couldn't open my right eye because it was swollen badly. If I opened my eyes, the pain got worse. For a couple of weeks, I could only see very little due to both eyes swelling shut. My right was the worst. I took Ibuprofen to feel better. I refused to let people take pictures of my face at that time because I continued to be embarrassed. Now, I regret not letting them because this experience was huge for me to be able to share. I tried to be brave and went to watch my team play their other games to support them.

During that summer and the first weeks of 6th grade, I went to therapy to heal my face. I also had to wear a couple of bandages. Students asked me what happened, so I explained to them the accident. In my 6th grade school year picture, it showed my scar-softball laces. My cheek still looked swollen, but I was feeling better. I also started wearing glasses because the accident impaired my vision. In my opinion, I looked great in my glasses. Looking on the bright side, at least I got to wear glasses out of the experience.

I wasn't going to give up on softball just yet. I decided to sign up for 4-H softball. I played softball in the summers of 2006 and 2007. It was a lot of fun and I got to play with some of my cousins. My favorite position continued to be pitching. One night I was pitching and a batter hit a line drive that ended up smacking my right hip bone. I went down to the ground, and I worried that it was broken. Luckily, it was not broken, but I did sit out of the game for a while. My cousin Zach told me that the batter laughed at me which made me feel even worse. After the summer of 2007, I made a decision to not play softball anymore. The injuries were hard for me to handle, and I still have a fear of getting hurt. Once we had to play softball in physical education class, and I kept worrying about getting hurt.

Throughout the years, I have learned a lot about how I think. I am not sure if other people with autism think the same way or not. For me, memories that are traumatic are clear and don't fade. I can remember every detail and the emotion that I was having at the time. However, the flashbacks of certain events hurt me more than others. This memory doesn't hurt me anymore because the physical pain went away. Plus, my family and friends showed me how much they loved me and cared for me.

Chapter Thirty-Four
Digging Deep with my Feelings
By Brittany Moreland, Lindsey's sister

Growing up as Lindsey's sibling, I never liked to share the things about autism that made me upset because I knew Lindsey couldn't help it, and I didn't like conflict. However, it is impossible to keep feelings inside forever. Just because your sibling has autism, doesn't mean everything you feel or do is related to autism.

When I was in 6th grade, Lindsey and I started staying home together for short periods of time while my mom was finishing up work. I was diagnosed with epilepsy in 4th grade which brought on a whole separate list of challenges for not only my family, but also me. My epilepsy was not a concern with regards to us staying home without our parents because my dad was only five minutes away, and Lindsey knew how to call him and had been taught how to help me in case I had a seizure.

In my eyes, I was the older daughter, so I felt the need to be in charge. When Lindsey wasn't listening to my directions, I would tell her to stop and also used sign language to help her understand that I meant she needed to stop. She hated this. She would push my hands away and start hitting herself, yelling and screaming. Her actions made me feel like I was the *bad sister*. I would apologize to make her stop hitting herself. After we cried together and hugged (always a deep pressure hug, a therapy technique that worked for Lindsey), we would go back to our normal routine. This happened often, and I was always the one giving in and apologizing. I felt guilty and felt that I was the cause of her actions. In the rest of my friendships and with family, I put the blame on myself and assumed that I was the cause of other people's problems, actions, and feelings.

This is a horrible way to feel and a cycle that's hard to break. I often wondered if other people who had siblings with special needs felt the same. I didn't know how to talk to anyone about it. I didn't know how to reach out for help. Years would pass by, and I continued to feel this way.

My 7th grade year was absolute hell! I was on several medications for my seizures. I was pretty much spaced out all of the time. Every little twitch and shake made me more worried about having a Grand Mal seizure. I spent more time in the nurse's office than in the classroom. I began losing my friends. They didn't know how to handle my problems, and I didn't know how to hide how awful I felt. I could feel classmates staring at me as my face twitched. They would laugh at me behind my back. No one knew what to do with me. I was not a behavior problem. I was stuck in the middle. The teachers acted annoyed with me. When it came to Lindsey, as soon as people heard that she had autism, she was adored by the teachers. Others tell me that this is "just" my perception, and yes, it is my perception and very real to me.

I know Lindsey didn't feel like she had real friends, but I didn't have friends, and I didn't have any teachers that appeared to be on my side or even wanted to relate to what I was going through. Trying to hold back tears each day and throughout the day was not successful. I cried at school, and I cried at home. Sometimes, I even cried on the bus.

Weighted down with all of my worries, I felt no purpose in my life. I was worthless in my mind and not worthy of being here on Earth. I couldn't meet others' expectations or live up to the challenges of school and family. I couldn't get out of bed, and wished I could be gone. If I couldn't be gone, I wished to be prettier, smarter, and more capable of handling life.

The words that echoed in my mind included the following phrases: "You are not smart enough," "You are not social enough," "You are not pretty enough," "Why are you here?" "What's the point?" and "You are a lost cause." I often asked, "What is God's plan?" I felt that I couldn't get any stronger. I questioned, "Why God are you doing this to me?"

Meanwhile, I was going to therapy as a part of Lindsey's therapy because my mom had recognized how sad I was with life. The therapist thought that my feelings were solely about Lindsey having autism. That was not the case. She gave my family odd strategies about letting me win in a game and letting me feel special. She also let me feel sorry for myself.

My depression was not related to having a sibling with autism. As an adult, I recall blaming my feelings and problems on others. I thought the cause of my pain was the actions of others rather than mine. In 7th grade, I spent fourteen days in the hospital for seizures. At that time, I was diagnosed with clinical depression.

As a teenager, I started wanting to be by myself and didn't want to hang out with Lindsey as much. I would be jamming out to my music, and Lindsey would be standing in the corner by my door, there waiting for me to notice her. She would ask if we could hang out. I would tell her that I wanted to be by myself.

Soon, she would start to cry and say, "It's alright...you don't want to be with me. I can be all alone. It's alright you don't like me." She would run to her room. Of course, I felt bad. I was dealing with more than typical teenage feelings and more than feelings due to Lindsey's autism.

Because I was dealing with clinical depression and didn't have the energy to hang out let alone get out from underneath the covers, I asked my mom to explain to Lindsey why I wanted to be by myself. The tables turned when Lindsey was a teenager. I did enjoy hanging out with her. Surprisingly, my sister put a special sign just for me on her door. It was a message about NOT disturbing her while she was doing homework because she was obsessed with not wanting to fail school.

As far as with friends and family, I truly believed that there were different expectations for me. When I was struggling with depression and Lindsey helped me by starting my car, packing my lunch, or even helping me wake up, I was judged as being lazy or not trying. However, when I helped Lindsey with anything it was ok because she had autism. As a sibling of a child with autism, I sometimes felt that the autism gave her permission to not understand or behave differently.

When I was young, I wanted to be on the television show *American Idol*. I told my mom I was a good singer and wanted to go on the show. She told me you wouldn't be good enough. She said she was sorry, but didn't want to lie. Years later, Lindsey was really into singing and she told my mom she wanted to go on *American Idol*. My mom said she would be great. I was puzzled because in my opinion Lindsey was pitchy sometimes. I asked my mom what was different and she said, "You could handle the truth."

When it came to talking about careers and choices after high school, the way my sister and I were treated differently was once again disappointing for me. I felt like my parents supported Lindsey in any decision she made. She told them that she wanted to work at a music store. Then, it changed to Spanish major, a teacher, etc. I wanted to be a physical therapist, but my parents said that the schooling would be too hard for me, so I researched other possibilities. The next day, I showed my mom the technical college I wanted to attend to become a cosmetologist. She laughed at me and said, "You have to do your own hair before you do someone else's hair." That whole summer I tried to prove her wrong. I always felt like I was trying to prove myself to everyone. Did Lindsey have to prove herself? Maybe she did, but not in the way that I felt like I was trying to prove myself.

The school system treated me differently, too. I had seizures, depression, and an eating disorder, but I didn't have autism. They didn't know what to do with me, but with Lindsey they tried to make everything right. When Lindsey was in high school, and she wasn't invited to prom, she told me that she was going to have her own prom at our house and post it on *Facebook*. Worried for her, I told her kids would make fun of her and that was not a good idea. I even told her that I would go to prom with her. After that, Lindsey wrote a scary message on Facebook about how she felt about not getting to go to prom. The school tried to make it right. They asked a classmate of Lindsey's to go to prom with her. I was so happy for her. I colored her hair, did her makeup, got the dress, and made sure it was the happiest weekend of her life. As happy as I was for her, I felt a little jealous. Was that all I had to do was post something bad on *Facebook* for someone to hear me?

In the summer of 2009, I had just finished my junior year of high school when I had another long hospital stay. Once again I had all of those electrodes hocked up to my head and some on other parts of my body. In the end it was determined that I was not having electrical seizures at that time. The shaking I was having in my legs was diagnosed as restless leg syndrome caused by an iron deficiency. I was also told that the seizure activity I was having in my face and hands was most likely due to anxiety and stress. I was excited and determined to turn my life around.

Due to my seizures and depression, I eventually got help through a program called D.V.R. (Division of Vocational Rehabilitation) which helped me get and keep a job. One time a client at my work stopped breathing and fell to the ground. I was the receptionist, and they told me to call 911. I froze because I didn't know the address to tell 911 where the salon was located. I started to have a panic attack. The job coach had to run over and take the phone, and also had to follow me home to make sure I was safe to drive. I felt terrible and embarrassed because I didn't know what to do. My brain could be on point, but any moment it could just all go away, and I would feel lost.

How is all this important to Lindsey's story? I choose to share it because I want other families to understand that siblings of children with autism may also have their own physical and emotional situations that they are dealing with layered onto the autism label the family wears each day.

Chapter Thirty-Five

"Affection for Adventure"

By Lauri Moreland, Lindsey's mom

It breaks my heart to hear and read Brittany's perception of her growing up years and how terrible she felt. Yet, I am glad she is able to express her thoughts, and that we have a great relationship today. The open communication has helped both of us. I never imagined I would have had even one child with special needs, let alone two. At times Brittany's epilepsy and its side effects were more difficult than Lindsey's autism. Brittany had several different therapists and finding the right one was not easy. Did I make mistakes in how I talked to her? Of course. My dad always says, "I did the best job I could raising you kids. You will take what you like and do it the same with your kids. What you didn't like, you won't do....and you will be the best parent." I truly did the best job I could do at the time considering our circumstances.

When Brittany and Lindsey were in middle school, I would come home exhausted from a long day's work and immediately Brittany would be chattering away about her next dream. It was never that I was giving up on her or didn't believe in her, I was simply exhausted.

I think that Brittany's excitement for adventure has always impressed me, but this has also made me want to protect her from disappointment. She was the kind of kid growing up that if she set her mind to something, she would figure out a way to do it, and she has. She has skydived. She got her cosmetology license. She has been both a clothing model and a hair model. She is a *Zumba* instructor, has taken multiple classes in cooking, painting, and salsa dancing, and is currently taking drum lessons. She ran a half marathon. She even went on a hunting trip with her dad and shot a bear. The bear rug hanging on the wall downstairs, the pictures, and the videos are all reminders of her affection for adventure. I am certain she has many more adventures in her future. She is a determined, strong-willed woman. She even has a tattoo on her rib that says, "Believe" as a symbol to herself to always believe in herself regardless of what she has overcome and what may lie ahead of her. Her dad and I weren't big fans of her getting a tattoo at the time, but we respect her confidence and beliefs.

Brittany talks about how she was treated differently from Lindsey when she expressed interest in pursuing something. This is absolutely 100% true. When Brittany said she wanted to be a physical therapist, I knew what it would take for this to happen. At the time she talked about this, she was having seizures and couldn't even make it through a whole school day. I was trying to be realistic, and I thought I was making the right decision by telling her how I felt. I was trying to spare her from failure. The doctors gave us a sheet of paper with at least fifteen different medical conditions or labels which included not only a seizure disorder but also attention deficit, depression, eating disorder, a learning disability, obsessive compulsive disorder, and anxiety disorder. Bottom line, I just wanted her to make it through a day of school without going to the nurse and being sent home. I wanted her to graduate high school. I could barely get her out of bed each day. Therefore, I shared my honest thoughts with her. I never intended to hurt her in anyway.

The difference between Lindsey's interests in singing on *American Idol* and Brittany's is that Lindsey would mention it once or twice, but then she wouldn't bring it back up. Brittany was relentless. I knew she wouldn't let it go until I bought plane tickets and flew her to an audition. So, I told her what I thought about her singing. What I saw on the show was people getting ripped apart and laughed at. I didn't want Brittany to have to go through something like that. I wasn't trying to imply that she wasn't a good singer, but I didn't think her level of singing was going to go professional.

When she talks about becoming a cosmetologist and my comments to her, I did say, "You have to learn how to do your own hair before you do anyone else's." I was frustrated that our morning routines were not going well. I could hardly wake her up, she would ask me to wash her hair, and most of the time walk out the door with wet hair, barely getting to school on time. This wasn't just for a day or two. This was all of her school years. When she was 17 years old, she was able to go off of all seizure medicine but continued to suffer from the side effects of seizures.

Looking back, I don't know how I survived. Most nights I sat on Brittany's bed side as she cried, trying to comfort her. I hugged her and rubbed her back. I was always trying to find the right words. There were nights that I sat with her until 11:00 p.m. Then, I had to get up at 5:00 in the morning to get ready to work. I worked 10 to 12 hour days at the time and had multiple phone calls a day from numerous different people, ranging from teachers, therapists, and doctors concerning both girls. Adding on to those calls, were calls from my clients and the paperwork of being self-employed. I was trying to keep it all together, plus do the daily household jobs of a mom...making meals, cleaning, and laundry. I also wanted to be a good wife. Todd and I had very little time together. He was working second shift and often was working on building projects at home. It seemed that when Brittany was anxious to tell me something, I was busy. In the perfect world I could have been a full time mom and not worked. That was really not an option.

I am proud of Brittany's perseverance and determination to be a successful adult. She has a bright future ahead of her with many more adventures.

Chapter Thirty-Six

"Being a pencil artist is my gifted talent."

By Lindsey Moreland

When I was in fourth grade, I wanted to be a singer. In fifth grade, I wanted to be a nurse. In sixth grade, I wanted to be a cop, and in seventh grade, I wanted to be an artist. Like the other kids my age, I looked around and was influenced by what I saw and heard. When I wanted to be a singer, I watched *American Idol* on television. I liked the auditions, but I also liked seeing who would win. Now, I listen to music for fun, love singing karaoke on my sister's karaoke machine, and in public with my sister. I don't want to be a professional singer anymore.

My inspiration in wanting to be a nurse came from the show *Untold Stories of the E.R.* I thought the stories were interesting and was fascinated by the doctors and how they performed the surgeries. When I realized I couldn't stand blood anymore, I knew that I wasn't going to be a nurse. Moving on to wanting to be a cop, it was the show *Cops*, the reality show, that inspired me. I thought it was entertaining watching them arrest people. Now, I do not want to be a cop. My dad told me it would be a dangerous job for me. You might say that television influenced me in many different ways.

However, not all of my influences came from television. In seventh grade, I got to take Spanish class. I liked learning a different language, and I thought it was unique. My teacher complimented me on how well I was learning Spanish. I don't know why, but I feel like Spanish is easier for me than English sometimes. This began my interest in other foreign languages. I checked out books from the library and bought books from the bookstore on French, Italian, Spanish, Chinese, Hindi, Japanese, and German. My parents continued to encourage my changing interests which made me grateful. Of all the languages, though, Spanish became a passion and something that I continue to speak today.

In middle school, we had student clubs on Fridays. Because I had gotten a good grade on a 3-D building I had done in art class in sixth grade, I decided to join an art club. During that time, I realized that I not only enjoyed pencil drawing, but I was also getting good at it. My confidence in my talent was building, and I wanted to sell my drawings. It was 2007, and I was 13 years old. Other kids might have been selling lemonade outside their house on a summer day, but not me. My sign that I artistically made read, "Art for Sale." The lowest price was $25, and the highest price was $65. I don't know what I was thinking, but I thought I would give it a try. Standing outside for half an hour, only one car stopped. It was one of my neighbors. They told me that they couldn't afford my drawings, but they thanked me for sharing it with them. Well, I gave it a shot! Today, I find this story funny. At the time, I was puzzled as to why no one would buy my drawings. My parents believed I could do anything and didn't discourage me from trying. I think they laughed a little, though.

Apparently, my teachers were also noticing my talent with my art. My middle school art teacher sent two projects of mine to the local art show in New Richmond, Wisconsin. One of the projects was called "Watercolor Illusion" and was of flower lilies. The other project was a batik project which is a wax resist, fabric color dying process. It was of a parrot. This success in art furthered my desire to continue being an artist.

I was part of a 4-H club. For three years, I entered my drawings at the county Fair. My drawings were mostly of animals. In 2008, my drawing of a collie received a top blue prize. In 2009, I decided it would be my last time to enter my drawings because it was very difficult for me to go in front of the judges and listen to their harsh criticism.

Each year, when it was time to bring my drawings to the fair, I would get nervous. Feeling the tension all over my body, I would sometimes even shake and sweat. At the fair, each person entering a drawing would have to stand in line and wait their turn to have their drawing be judged. Talking to the judge about my art wasn't too hard for me, but I was afraid that what they would say to me would hurt my feelings. One time, the judge didn't like the detail on the fur of a cheetah drawing I had made. I had looked at a picture of a cheetah and drew it exactly like the picture. As an artist, I feel like I can draw it the way I see it, but not everyone may see it the same way that I do.

In high school, my art teacher was impressed with my work and had a way to be both respectful of my perspective and helpful at the same time. I appreciated her thoughts and advice for my art. In my freshman and junior years, my artwork was displayed in the lobby for one of the best artworks of the year.

In a previous chapter where I talked about my fascination with *Titanic,* I mentioned that *Titanic* was one of my favorite subjects to draw. I couldn't stop myself from wanting to draw the ship in the last years of middle school. Assigned projects in high school and other commitments prevented me from having the time to draw the *Titanic* in high school. As an adult, I first drew the *Titanic* again at the age of 21. After drawing it, my passion for it resumed. I started thinking about it from different angles, perspectives, and situations. My current drawings of it include the sinking of it, the landscapes, different rooms in the ship such as the grand staircase, and the striking of the iceberg. I have learned a lot about how my brain works when it comes to my passions. When I start something I am passionate about, I think about it every day. For example, when it came to drawing, I would plan out when I would draw and see if my mood felt like it was a good day for me to draw. In addition to drawing the *Titanic,* I have begun to draw many places around the world, celebrities, and objects. When I draw, I either draw what interests me from a picture I have seen or a place I want to travel someday. Using the picture as a model helps me not miss anything as I add every detail including the shadowing.

September 12th, 2015 was a Saturday, and my mom, my sister, and I went to see Art on the River, an art display tradition in a local town. At the art display, I could visualize myself selling my art someday. Once a week, I would go online to the chamber of commerce to see the applications for 2016. When applications were available, I printed one out and showed my mom. I was excited and thought it would be a good opportunity. Unfortunately, while being a full-time college student, it was not the right time.

While selling my art is a way to feel successful, displaying my art in public was a bigger dream of mine. The same town also had a Main Street art festival on October 17, 2015. This was similar to the Art on the River. There, I met many different artists. One of the artists talked to me and told me about the Wisconsin Regional Art Program (WRAP). This would be a chance to display my drawings. The exhibit was located at the gallery in the basement of the local public library. A couple days later, I received information about the program and the limit of submitting three pieces of artwork. When it was January, 2016, I had to choose the artwork from my extensive collection of drawings that I had been working on for a year. What a tough decision! How would I ever choose? I love all of my drawings, and I am proud of them. Choosing a *Titanic* drawing made sense and was easy for me. The other two drawings I chose were "The First Class Grand Staircase" and a portrait of Amy Winehouse, a deceased rhythm and jazz blues singer from London, England. I chose to draw Amy Winehouse because she is one of my favorite singers of all time. She had a raspy, blues voice and a lot of talent. Plus, I dressed up as her for Halloween, 2015. On January 30, 2016, I paid a small fee and entered my three drawings. Upon entering them, the employer at the gallery mentioned how much she loved the drawings. She said that pencil drawings were one of the art mediums that were hardly displayed in the past year of the program. The 2nd annual WRAP Exhibit went from February 6th to March 5th, 2016.

Displaying my drawings in public for others to see was a dream come true. On opening day, I went to the exhibit with my roommate Greta. I couldn't believe it! My art pieces were there-right at the entry of the gallery. How exciting! Not only that, I was the only artist who displayed pencil drawings. Most of the other artwork was pottery, painting, and jewelry. On February 13, 2016, judges looked at the work and awarded honorable mentions and work that qualified to win for the state. Thankfully, I did not have to go in front of the judges like I did in 4-H. What was most important to me was that my artwork was included in the art show. Without having to meet the judges, I didn't have to feel the tension or pressure of having to win something. At 2:00 p.m. that day, the judges would announce winners. I arrived at 1:00 p.m. to meet other artists from the show. Fourteen winners were announced and fourteen others received honorable mention. My name wasn't mentioned. Awards are nice, but they are not the reason why I wanted to display my drawings. Sharing my work with others means a lot to me. I feel like it shows them a little bit of who I am and what I can do. I believe all people have talents and should be brave enough to share them.

My family was proud of me and continues to be proud of me. They help me and support me regardless of what I want to do. Whenever I tell my mom, my dad, or my sister that I want to do something, they say, "This is a wonderful idea." When I told my mom I wanted to enter my artwork she said, "Go for it," and I did. To be supportive, my parents came to the show February 13th, the day of the award ceremony. My sister Brittany came on the last day of the exhibit, March 5, 2016. Brittany thought that my *Titanic* drawing should have won state. I thanked her for her honesty, but I am completely happy how everything turned out. I was glad my uncle Bob went to see it, too. He saw it on February 13, 2016. He even took a picture of it and sent it to me on my phone. When family members support me, I express my gratitude to them. This is my true award.

I loved the experience so much that I didn't want it to end. Wishing it would have lasted longer than a month so that other relatives and friends could have seen it, I knew that it would be ok because I plan on entering artwork again in the following years. Drawing continues to be a favorite hobby of mine. Currently, I am drawing more and will have to decide which ones to display next.

In 2017, I participated in WRAP again. I didn't get any awards, but I'm completely proud of my accomplishments. I received an exciting opportunity to display my drawings locally at a winery in Wisconsin. I have always dreamed of displaying my drawings locally, and my dreams have come true! I can finally check it off from my bucket list! The opening day at the winery was wonderful. A couple of my drawings were sold, and some of the proceeds went to *Autism Speaks*.

I entered my drawings for a couple silent auctions in an annual art show at a local school. All of my drawings sold! Because my drawings were displayed and were entered in art shows and silent auctions, I designed my own business cards and *Facebook* page: "Lindsey Moreland-Pencil Artist." The website for my page is https://www.facebook.com/lindseymoreland2/.

I would rather be drawing and listening to music for fun than dealing with singing auditions, audiences booing at my music, and exhausting tours. I would rather be drawing than dealing with graphic wounds and blood even if it meant helping people. I would rather be drawing than dealing with traffic stops or helping keep the world safe. All occupations and hobbies are important, but this is the right one for me.

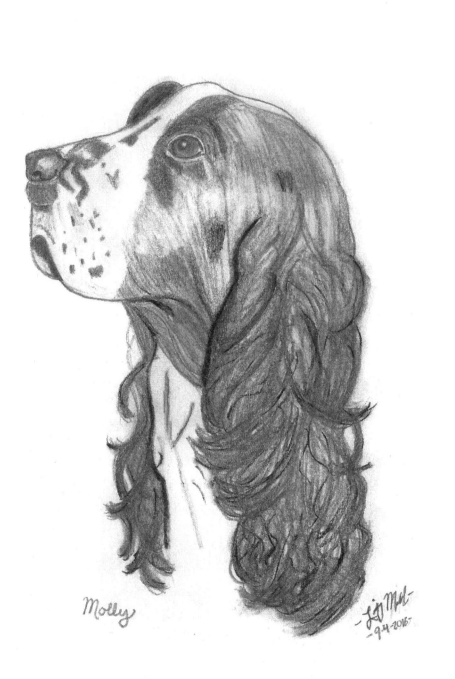

Molly

LizMit
9-4-2016

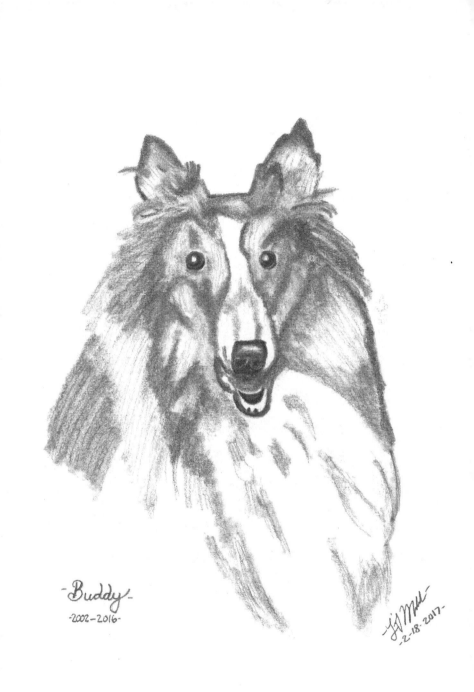

-Buddy-
-2002-2016-

149

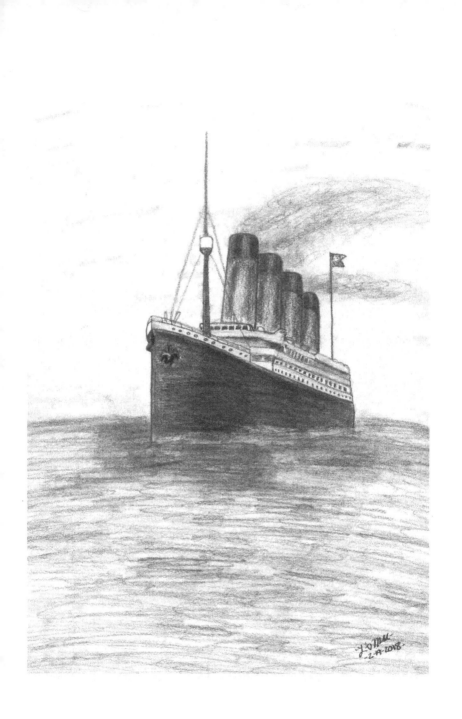

Chapter Thirty-Seven
"Her friends were her family."
By Lauri Moreland, Lindsey's mom

Lindsey made it through middle school, but she still didn't have any friends. Her teachers continued to be her friends. As she entered high school, once again, I hoped and prayed that this would be her year to make some lasting friendships. I also hoped Brittany would start feeling better about herself. I felt fortunate that our girls got along most of the time and always had each other.

As a family, we enjoyed many happy adventures. We loved spending time out on the lake paddle boating, fishing, and swimming. We took a few vacations as well. We went to California and Florida twice. We loved spending time together in our log home. I felt like we had come so far as a family with a child with autism. Lindsey was able to communicate with us and was now functioning at a high level. She had, and has, a unique way of seeing the world. She had us laughing and questioning how we use language in our everyday lives.

One day we were on the paddleboat with a friend, and the friend used the expression, "You must be pooped." Lindsey's response was, "My mom not poop." She loved telling jokes, but she always prefaced it with, "I am going to tell you a joke, and you can laugh." She recognized details, especially the size of people. She told her grandpa's friend that he had a big belly. We were embarrassed, but his wife did thank Lindsey when he lost fifteen pounds on a diet. When she was little, I prayed she would talk. When she got older, I prayed that what she would say would be nice and appropriate. The older she got, it was less appropriate for her to say some of the things that she was saying. In middle school, she pointed out the size of people's legs right to their face. At a restaurant, she told a customer that "smoking is naughty." When we were selling our car, she asked the prospective buyer, "Why do you want to buy our blue bomber?" She even went so far as to call a stranger's car a brown bomber because the paint was peeling off of the car just like the blue car that we owned. Teaching her to notice without commenting was something we worked on with her. She was comfortable saying what she was thinking when she was around us, but not in school. I wondered if she had been more comfortable talking in school if she would have had friends.

Lacking positive experiences at school, we tried our best to make our home life exciting, happy, relaxing, comforting, and fun. We continued water therapy, deep pressure, and other sensory therapy. We enjoyed inviting friends and family to our house. Lindsey did well most of the time. If she got overwhelmed, she would take a break in her room. It was much easier for people to come to us, but we always attended family gatherings. As Lindsey got older, she also got more comfortable around her cousins and family friends. She even looked forward to fun times with them because they treated her well and understood how autism affected her interactions with them. They knew when to include her, when to let her have her own space, and time alone. They always invited her to participate and continued to try even if she declined.

In high school, she was shy. She had an extreme fear of being late to class and getting good grades. She focused her attention on studying. I knew that she struggled to make eye contact, but she never told me that people were laughing or making fun of her. I found out from my nephew, who went to the same high school, that Lindsey sat alone each day at lunch. How could the teachers not notice? Why wouldn't kids sit by her? I remember all of Lindsey's IEP meetings well and have spent hours looking over years of Individualized Education Plans. Every report states that Lindsey had peer difficulties and "did not appear to have close friends." Specifically, one IEP reads, "Lindsey has difficulty developing friendships among peers because she lacks many of the social skills that are necessary for interaction." Although I voiced my concerns and suggested starting a "Circle of Friends" group for Lindsey and any other students who might benefit from it, it was never started. Brittany would come home crying about school, but Lindsey never told me that she was sad about school. Years later, she told me that she would come home and cry in her bedroom. I thought she was studying or needed her alone time.

The year after Lindsey graduated, we often thought about how we could help others and make a difference. Lindsey had given a persuasive speech in a college speech class advocating for the prevention of bullying. I had already been asked several times to speak to educators and families about our experience with autism. Families and educators wanted to know what worked for us. We knew that there were other students out there like Lindsey who were missing out on school friendships, school activities, and being bullied. It was brought to our attention that a student on the autism spectrum was struggling in her junior year of high school. She wanted friends, but she didn't feel like she had any. Lindsey and I got involved. We met with her principal. At this time, I shared my disappointment with him that Lindsey never had a "Circle of Friends" group. He sincerely listened, and we began communicating with him on how to start a program. Both Lindsey and I offered to volunteer to help. Lindsey gave a speech to the students and a speech to the staff. We were overwhelmed and proud that the school implemented S.O.S (Students Offering Support). Several years have gone by, and the communication we have received about it is positive. I highly encourage not only parents of children with autism, but all parents to talk to their school district about having a program that supports the development of friendships.

Chapter Thirty-Eight

The Pageant

Introduction: By Linda Wagner, Lindsey's aunt

Here it is chapter thirty-eight, and there has never been an introduction to a chapter. When I began helping the Moreland family tell their story through the writing of this book, I never intended to be a part of any chapter. I understood my role in this project. I would meet with each family member, listen to their story, and then help get the words on paper that truly reflected their memories. Lindsey typically has written all of her chapters before we have met. When we would meet, we would go over the chapters together making a few minor adjustments.

When Lindsey sent me this chapter about running for town royalty (town ambassadors), I was confused by it because it didn't feel like the writing I would typically get from her. It bothered me, and I knew why. It was Wednesday, June 28, 2017 when I asked Lindsey to write this chapter. I had been over at her house working with Lauri on a chapter, and it was clear that Lindsey was not having a good day. Before we started writing, we sat with Lindsey on the porch. We talked with her as she sipped coffee and tried to hold back the tears. She apologized many times for feeling the way she was feeling. Reminding her that she could feel any way she wanted or needed, we did our best to help her feel better.

Lindsey had been searching for a job as a paraprofessional in school districts near her house. She had two successful interviews, however, a different candidate was chosen. This was upsetting to all of us. If someone could just give Lindsey a chance, she would be an excellent employee. Lindsey had volunteered in two different schools and both schools loved her! Lindsey had volunteered in my classroom multiple school years. All of the children adored her. They would make her cards, bring her gifts, and often begged to work with her. One of the parents of a student with autism even credits Lindsey for her child's success during the school year. She is the kindest, most empathetic person that has ever stepped foot into my classroom.

Upon reading The Pageant chapter over and over again, I kept getting more and more upset. I knew that when Lindsey wrote this she was discouraged, full of anxiety and stress over the job situation, and still she was trying to stay as positive as possible with this chapter. While Lindsey knows she continues to work on her grammar, this is typically not how she writes. Initially, I called Lauri and told her, "We need to fix this chapter." We talked about Lindsey's state of mind at the time and how when things are upsetting for her, it affects her ability to communicate the way she typically communicates. So, we decided to talk to her about changing it a bit, fixing the grammar, and taking out the negative. We wanted a happy chapter. Bottom line, we both wanted a happy Lindsey.

A couple of days passed when I felt like someone had thrown a brick right at my stomach. I sat down by my computer, and I cried and cried. How dare I try to fix this chapter? How dare I try to convince Lindsey to change the way she felt that day and her memories of the pageant? How dare I try to fix Lindsey to make myself feel better-like we were all trying to do? Lindsey is perfect exactly the way God has made her. She is the sweetest, kindest, most respectful person in the world. She is talented, smart, an excellent daughter, sister, niece, friend, and girlfriend. On top of that, she changes lives for the better. This may be the best chapter you read because it is untouched in any way.

Finally, it is a reminder for all of us on how Lindsey's autism displays itself in her adult years. When Lindsey is having a tough day, brought on by different factors, her communication skills are affected.

The Pageant

By Lindsey Moreland

Starting middle school, I **want** to be involved in sports and plays. When I was in 5th and 6th grade, I was in plays. In the **summer, before** going to 6th grade, I joined softball, but unfortunately, I was involved in an accident. During play practices, I was taking it seriously so teachers wouldn't be annoyed. **When there are students who were joking around and makes teachers impatient, I feel embarrassed.** Not only that, I also feel embarrassed when there are students who **ignored** me, treated me poorly, and laughed behind my back. In 7th grade, I decided not to join sports or plays because I didn't want to be with students who were mean to me.

When it comes to high school, again, I hardly joined clubs, sports, or plays because of **my safety towards mean students.** I also didn't want to participate because I was **worried for my homework** assignments and studying for upcoming tests. If there **wasn't** too **much** studies to worry about, then I would've joined school-related events. In sophomore year, I decided to sign up for the local pageant **to be town royalty** and an ambassador for my town.

In the winter, I received **a mail** about participating in it. I wasn't sure about it at first **because of all the process** it takes during the school year. I decided I would join because I **hope** to be an extrovert and hang out with friends. **After thinking about it, I was having thoughts of being in the paper if I get on court, the dress, the commercials based on what I sponsored.** I was excited **that I shared** my news to family members at the 50th wedding anniversary party. They seemed impressed.

On the first day, we had a meeting with the court, **and other candidates with their mothers about what the pageant is all about. 15** other girls in my class were **participating, that's the most they have throughout the years!** We would **be at** after school practices weekly, find our silver and gold sponsors, selli**ng** candles, selli**ng** roses, participat**ing** in two parades, and havi**ng** a couple parties with the court.

In the process of doing a commercial, I thought about what sponsors I should do. My gold sponsor was a credit union, and my silver sponsor was a coffee shop. I thought about doing a parody song of Beyoncé's "Single Ladies." Instead of singing "all the single ladies", I sang "All you Town Folks!" The first verse I did was about the credit union, and the second verse was about the coffee shop. I decided to dress in black and have a long black glove with the biggest ring on my finger. I would also do the dance moves, similar to Beyoncé. Since this is one of her popular songs, I thought this would be a great, fun way to do the advertising of the commercial.

During the first couple weeks of practicing, the candidates, myself included were selling candles. The candidate with the most sales will get a prize at the pageant show. **I thought I had the most sales, but I came in second, off by a couple of points. But I did receive a prize, which was the gift card.**

I did **found** the dress that I would wear for the pageant, and I got it from Macy's. **It was a long teal colored mermaid dress.** The candidates and I wore our dresses for the first day of practice and dress rehearsals. On the first day, I found out that I was contestant #4.

As far as this goes, I dealt with people who I'm terrified **with**. One of the girls **in** court was extremely bossy and crabby. Sometimes, she asked the candidates to pay attention and be quiet in a harsh manner. I **get** embarrassed and annoyed. She constantly reminded us to remember to smile and tells us our do's and don'ts. I didn't want her near me during those practices, even though she was kind to me and understands my autism. I didn't understand why her attitude had to be so poor. **The day before the pageant, we were serving food to people, she's still bossy and crabby, wanting us to do our best.She** made me cry while I was cleaning up the place. **I tried to hide it but the candidates did see me sad, but I couldn't tell anyone because I didn't want to make her feel bad.** But at the same time, I didn't want her to have anything to do with me. In freshman year, she did **made** fun of me in one of the classes for not doing well **in** one stupid quiz. It was also one of the classes where intelligent students **don't do well and the ones who weren't intelligent, ended up doing well in a quiz.** It really doesn't make sense. After the pageant, she was positive and said to me that I did an excellent job and had a great time working with me. If she had a great time, then why be so rude and bossy constantly?

There was **one in court** who was really nice to me and we would talk a lot. She knew my autism and **she has been given** me chances. The other two girls in court were also nice, even though they didn't talk to me much. The candidates were sometimes friendly, but not all of them though. During **partiesl,** they wouldn't even **asked** me to do something with them. Part of my autism is that I **was** afraid to ask them to hang out with me because I get anxious for being rejected. **That's why at first I just stand there to hang** out and watch other people talk to each other. I just wait until I finally get the conversation with them.

Other than trying to socialize, I was trying to have a great experience. The candidates had to write about themselves for the Town paper, and mine was short and simple. We also had to submit our baby pictures so readers **can** guess what **baby picture belongs to**. The Saturday before Mother's Day, the candidates and I were selling roses outside and a lot of cars drove into **but** the roses. It **went** successful. The following Saturday, the candidates and I were **on** the parade in a neighboring town and later watch their town's pageant. There was only one incident. When I was in **Phy** Ed. **I** hurt my knee and I had to wear **a knee for** only a couple of days, including the day of practice. The day after the practice and wearing the knee brace, I passed my driver's license. **Silly as it sounds! The** week of the town celebration the candidates were helping out in tents, outside of the carnival. We also **help** serve food to people the day before the pageant.

On the day of the pageant, the candidates and I **were having** an interview with the judges. During the interview of each candidate, we had to vote for Miss Congeniality. After the interview, we had a tea party and later went **on** the parade. Each candidate rode on **the** convertible with the posters of their sponsors.

On the evening of the pageant, my aunts and uncles, my grandparents, my grandma from Iowa, my cousin, my parents, and Brittany came to this special event to support me. The candidates and I did a dance for "Walking on Sunshine." After the dance, each candidate walked down the aisle with their dads (or moms). Later on, each **candidate perform their commercials**. After that, each candidate walked around the stage with their gowns and answer one question. According to the question, **I answered about having a goal to help other families with autism and let others learn how to accept their differences.** When the crowning began, I won second place for the most sales in candles. There

will be four princesses and one queen. When third princess was announced, I thought I would get crowned by the girl (the third princess) who was standing behind me, but the crown was given to the girl next to **me.That** was close. I didn't get crowned on court, but I was excited for the candidates who were crowned. I was the only one who didn't cry because I was extremely happy how this turned out.

I'm kind of glad I didn't get **in** because I didn't want to hurt my cheeks for smiling all the time and spending gas prices for traveling to different places for parades. I would've missed out on the fun though. My family was extremely **proud of me how this turned out and** that I did an excellent job. The court and newly crowned candidates congratulated me on how well I did.

A month later, one of the girls who didn't get on court decided to throw a non-court party. It didn't make sense because there should've been a party including the girls who were crowned. One of the girls who **were** crowned was pissed off because she didn't get invited and that this entire idea of a non-court party was completely odd. I appreciated that I was invited and had fun, but at the same time, this was awkward.

After the pageant, I thought I would socialize and hang out with people, but I was very wrong. I **was stilled** ignored and treated poorly by students in junior and senior year. They wanted nothing to do with me. I felt hurt again. I hate to mention this, **but I had the right to feel that way and it isn't fair, but unfortunately, fair is fair**. I tried not to be hard on myself, but that's challenging when I felt like **a nobody**.

Chapter Thirty-Nine

"Chatting about the Pageant Experience"

By Lindsey Moreland and Lauri Moreland, Lindsey's mom

*Sitting in a freezing, air-conditioned coffee shop on a warm July day in 2017, this conversation was recorded between Lindsey and Lauri.

Lauri: I am grateful, Lindsey, that you were willing to keep chapter thirty-eight untouched. I know it was hard for you to reread it and not change grammar or sentence structure. Remember when you were changing the word "want" to "wanted," and we begged you to change it back to its original form? We hope Chapter thirty-eight helps others better understand communication difficulties with people who have autism.

Lindsey: I really wanted to change it. There are so many rules with grammar to remember, and it's hard to remember all of them and even harder when I am stressed out.

Lauri: Can we talk about the pageant experience?

Lindsey: Yes we may.

Lauri: I remember when you came home with the paper with the information about the pageant and you wanted to know what I thought and what Brittany thought about it. Both Brittany and I were excited and said, "Go for it." I was shocked because I never thought you would put yourself out there to do something like this. I immediately thought about taking you dress shopping.

Lindsey: I was thankful that you were going to allow me to participate in this exciting opportunity. The dress shopping put a smile on my face, and I was looking forward to trying on dresses too. So then we had to go to the informational, sign up meeting right mom? It was the first week in February.

Lauri: Yes, we went to the meeting together. Parents had to agree that if you did get on court, we would support you with all of the events. It also talked about what you had to wear, like two different dresses.

Lindsey: Mom, I knew you would be supportive no matter what. At the meeting, I looked around the room at the other girls. I counted 14 other girls, and I was looking to see who they were...I was hoping there wouldn't be any girls that were mean. I hoped to be treated well.

Lauri: I was watching you from afar. I wanted to see how you were interacting with the other girls. I noticed that you would be in the group, on the edge, and also standing a couple inches back. I was nervous. I wanted this to be the first good experience in high school.

Lindsey: Yes, I didn't know how to socialize well. That has been a part of my struggles all of my life. It is just not easy for me to know what to do.

Lauri: So, the four month adventure began. Weekly, you went to rehearsals. You were going to get to dance. I was excited to see you dance and be with the other girls. You still seemed a little uncomfortable, but it was clear that you were trying and really wanted to do well.

Lindsey: Yes!

Lauri: I remember the night that you were told that you had to sell candles to promote the town. Previously when you sold things for school, I typically just bought the items myself because it was easier and I didn't like you girls asking others for money. This time, however, I felt like both dad and I supported you a lot. We drove you around. We brought the order form to work. We had support from family and friends. It was more than selling candles. It was that we wanted you to win and be the top seller of the candles.

Lindsey: I remember I sold over $1,200 dollars' worth of candles. That was a lot of candles to sell and deliver. I was completely happy to get second place in candle sales, but mom you didn't seem too happy about it.

Lauri: That is only because I was told by someone involved with the pageant that you had the top sales for the candles. I was in shock that night when your name wasn't called.

Lindsey: I still got recognized and got a gift card to Target. We also had to sell roses. It was a park in town.

We sold them for Mother's Day. Each candidate had to be waving at cars. We had a poster. It was a windy day.

Lauri: That's right. I saw pictures of your hair just blowing.

Lauri: Let's talk about the fun time we had going shopping for your dress.

Lindsey: We went to Macy's. There were a lot of dresses. I tried on a handful of dresses before I found the one I really liked. The dress I chose was a strapless, teal, mermaid dress with a diamond like bead or brooch right where you could cover up cleavage.

Lauri: Not that you had much cleavage to cover up Lindsey. (Laughs) It did fit you like a glove, though.

Lindsey: (laughs) I was the only one in the pageant with a mermaid dress. I felt like myself in that dress. It was the right dress for me. Most of all, I just felt beautiful.

Lauri: Going into the shopping experience, I was prepared to spend whatever it took on the dress. I just wanted to make sure you felt like a million bucks.

Lindsey: I didn't want it to be over the top expensive. I found it on the clearance rack at Macy's.

Lauri: It was around 100 dollars.

Lindsey: It kind of looked new.

Lauri: Lindsey, it was new! (More laughs and smiles between both Lauri and Lindsey)

We were fortunate to borrow the second dress from a friend.

Lindsey: Yes, we had to wear the second dress for the town parade. Each candidate got to sit on the top of a convertible and ride in the parade. I got to ride on a car that belonged to my dad's co-worker. It was a silver Sebring convertible.

Lauri: I did your hair for the parade.

Lindsey: Yes, I had to sit there for over an hour getting my hair curled. I had to have patience.

Lauri: You sure came far from the screaming during haircuts and getting your hair brushed. It still hurt you, though.

Lindsey: Haircuts still hurt. My head is super sensitive....all the tugging and pulling is excruciating. I would like to put my hair up, but I can't do it. That's why I leave it down. I don't mind getting my hair curled. It's not as bad.

Lauri: I remember the day of the parade well. It was a cloudy, cool day, but we were all super excited. I remember exactly where we sat on Main Street right outside the bank. We screamed a lot when you rode by. Lindsey, you looked like a princess waving to the crowd. You seemed so happy. Do you remember us cheering for you and taking pictures?

Lindsey: I heard you. I did feel like a million bucks. The pageant was the same day as the parade. We also had a tea party.

Lauri: When you went to the tea party, we went home. How did you feel at the tea party?

Lindsey: It was ok, but all I could eat there was fruit because there was no gluten free food. At the tea party, you hang out with candidates along with previous court and current court from other towns.

Lauri: Did that make you have anxiety?

Lindsey: No, I felt really included.

Lauri: While you were at the tea party, your dad was home getting ready for the pageant. He had the honor of walking you down the aisle. All dads were going to be walking their daughters down the aisle of the auditorium. He had his sports coat on and dress pants. I knew he was proud of you.

Lindsey: Yeah, it was a great moment for dad and me to walk down together. We didn't get to wear one of our dresses. We had to wear an outfit from a second hand store. I wore a black shirt, jeans, a black hat, and a purse. I am thankful Dad would use his time to support me. Dad has given me great support all of my life.

Lauri: We had a lot of friends and family that attended and supported you, too. It was fun to see everyone there.

I remember sitting near the front row. A friend even video-taped it for us.

Lindsey: We came out and had fun with a group dance to the song, "Walking on Sunshine." Everyone said that I was smiling the most. I was told millions of times by one of the girls on court to remember to smile, and I did. She was kind of bossy about it. Not to be mean or rude or anything, but it was making me uncomfortable.

Lauri: When I saw you on stage, I was holding back the tears. It was a proud moment. Smiling had been so hard for you along with eye contact. Here you were smiling bigger and brighter than all of the other candidates. I am sure I am a little biased.

Lindsey: After that, I had so much fun sharing my commercial.

Lauri: I thought that you did a great job with it. It was cute and funny.

Lindsey: "All the Single Ladies" by *Beyoncé* was really popular at that time, so I thought it would be a great parody.

Lauri: I thought the whole night went great. You had a great answer to your final question. You wanted to support people who had autism. You weren't feeling bad about having autism, you were just real and matter of fact about it. I was proud of how great you answered the question.

Lindsey: I just thought of this today, mom. What I am doing now with my motivational speaking and writing this book is helping others better understand people with differences. This is what I wanted all along.

Lauri: Wow! These thoughts about helping people started way back when you were in tenth grade.

Lauri: I had really mixed feelings about the crowning of the queen and princesses. I thought you did just as well as all of the other candidates. You had a great attitude, a great commercial, and answered your question well. I did wonder how they picked the court. I wondered why they didn't give you a chance. However, I saw how happy you were which made me feel a lot better. I did feel a little relieved because I was in the state of mind of trying to protect you. How would you handle a summer of parades and how would you interact with the other girls?

Lindsey: I was the only one who didn't cry. You should talk about that.

Lauri: When it was over, all of the candidates went to the back room, and that is where I was to pick you up. All of the other candidates who didn't get on a court were crying and you were congratulating the girls that got on court. You were also telling the other girls that it was ok.

Lindsey: I was optimistic that whole time, and I was happy for them. Being the only girl not crying about it, made me feel brave.

Lauri: We drove home and we talked about it. You kept telling us that it was great. You also told us that we were going to save big bucks not having to drive all over the place.

Lindsey: I wouldn't have to be reminded to smile so much anymore.

Chapter Forty
"Dreams do come true."
By Lindsey Moreland

Why is it that I had friends in elementary school, and then they drifted away in middle and high school? In my senior year, just four weeks before graduation, I was in English Communications class and I had to interview and write about two other classmates. It truly hurts me because I was lonely and ignored, and I didn't know who to write about since other students already signed up to interview their friends.

At first, I thought I would interview one of the nicest students who respected and treated me well, even though we didn't socialize a lot. But when she rejected me, I felt betrayed, puzzled, and confused. The next day, Wednesday, April 25, 2012, I felt like someone stabbed me in the heart. When I was looking at the list of student names, I saw that the nice student accepted someone else to interview her. What did I do to make myself more isolated? After looking at the list, still seeing no name next to my name, I went to the restroom to let out my tears until they would dry on their own. At the same time, I wished I wasn't born so I wouldn't have to deal with this pain of having no friends.

Even though I felt like the teachers were my friends, there were days when I wondered if teachers pretended they liked me so they wouldn't have to deal with me and my autistic behaviors. I thought teachers in high school were going to set up the "Circle of Friends" program, just like elementary school, but they never did. I was ready to throw in the towel. I was so hurt by the terrible way I was treated and ignored. Enough is enough. I had enough of this mess. After feeling lonely and isolated, and not getting the help I needed, I decided to take a stand by sharing how I was feeling on *Facebook*. I didn't care if I got into trouble with my parents because I wanted others to understand what I was going through. I was sick and tired of not being accepted and not belonging anywhere. Here's what I wrote:

"Today or actually everyday has been bad for me. Throughout my stupid years of middle and high school, no one likes to be partners with me in every class, to hang out with me, go to sporting events, prom, or any other fun stuff with me, but WHATEVER! Everybody hates me. That's because I'm different. I guess people don't like others who are odd, different, but I had a heart, broken every year. I had it!! My goal was to have a great senior year, well that didn't happen!"

I didn't write this post to get attention, I just wanted people to know how I felt. People were worried and concerned about my situation. After some classmates read my post, they apologized. I thought it was going to take forever to accept their apologies because I was so hurt. I didn't respond right away because I was having mixed feelings at the same time. I just pressed the "Like" button. But I felt they really meant it, so I accepted their apologies.

The next day, April 26th, after school, I went home and my Mom told me that she did go to high school and had a private conversation with the principal about my *Facebook* post. He was sorry and wanted to help. But how, after only having four weeks left to graduate? Wasn't it a little too late for that? Later, my principal called Mom on the phone saying that a classmate, a popular and talented basketball player, was going to ask me to go to prom with him. It was truly unexpected and I was shocked. My Mom and I thought this was some kind of joke. That evening Brittany colored and cut my hair to look healthy for Saturday. I already had a dress because my sister was going to let me borrow the one she had worn in my cousin's wedding. I also found shoes and jewelry. This was short notice, but this type of short notice was a good thing.

It was Friday morning, and my name was announced to go to the office, so I went there. There he was, and he asked me to prom. Throughout that time, I was so grateful to him. I was almost in tears of happiness, but I had to hold them in so I wouldn't be embarrassed from others staring at me in the hallway. That was the only great school day I had, and I was much happier than I had been. When it was evening, I was getting ready for the big day. My sister was doing my nails.

It was Saturday, April 28, 2012, the day of prom. I woke up early in the morning at 5:30 because I was too excited to stay asleep. Brittany styled my hair for two hours. I was so thankful to her for everything she was doing to help me prepare for this special school event. Without her, I wouldn't know what I would look like. At 2:30 p.m. my date arrived at my log house with another prom couple. They were friendly and kind and most of all, respectful. Then, all of the parents were at the house for picture taking. We also had pictures out by a lake, and it was cold outside. Later, we drove to a candy shop for even more pictures.

My friends and I went to the *Mall of America* for dinner. We ate at "The Cadillac Ranch." After dinner, we went to *Build-A-Bear-Workshop*. I didn't expect to go there, but my date wanted me to have a bear for a special remembrance of prom, so he bought me one. After the mall, we went to get ice cream treats.

It was 8:00 in the evening when we went back for prom at the high school. It was loud, but it was worth it and enjoyable. The theme for prom was "Singing in the Rain." The theme was great because it was raining on that day. The designs in the gymnasium were cute, creative, and beautiful. We danced together only on fast songs. I was unexpectedly reunited with some friends I used to have, and they were glad to see me. If they're happy, I'm happy as well. Students actually talked to me and found out that I am a fun person. If only they would have been more educated about autism, maybe my school years could have been different. The grand march was at 10:00 p.m. My family was there to see me. There were many pictures taken throughout the grand march, and there were many smiles from everyone's faces. That impressed me the most because it tells me that they were sorry for the way they treated me. The principal mentioned, "I know it's a little and a little too late."

Around 11:00, close to midnight, I was dropped off at my home, and my date walked with me to the garage door. I definitely thanked him for the wonderful night, and he was also glad that he had fun.

Prom was like a fairy tale. Before my graduation ceremony, I finally socialized with other classmates. Not only prom was a dream come true, but graduating with honors was a dream of mine. At the end of my sophomore year, my sister graduated high school. I saw that there were students wearing golden ropes. I told my Mom one day that I wanted to buy one so I could wear it with my cap and gown. I didn't know it was something you earned by getting excellent grades and becoming an honor student. I was determined to work hard with my homework and study a lot for upcoming tests or finals. That's one of the reasons why I was an introvert.

My dream came true. I didn't have to buy it. A week before graduation, I was interviewed by a journalist about being a student with autism, graduating with honors. I wished my mom was there with me because she explains it better than I do in certain ways. I didn't like the title, "Lindsey Moreland Overcomes Autism by Graduating with Honors." First of all, I didn't agree because I can't overcome it. Second, autism doesn't go away. After graduating high school, I got accepted to a Wisconsin university for Spanish. I tested out of the first year of Spanish. I also got accepted to a technical College for generals. Last but not least, I received a scholarship from a credit union from my home town. I was even more proud of myself.

Chapter Forty-One
"Getting Involved"
By Lauri Moreland, Lindsey's mom

May 26, 2012, Lindsey graduated from high school. We were all proud of her. She had worked hard to graduate with honors. In elementary school, I was at school on a weekly basis and stayed in contact with her teachers. By middle school, I went there on a monthly basis and continued to communicate frequently with her teachers. When Lindsey was in high school, I wanted to respect what I believed to be age appropriate. Obviously, I wasn't eating lunch with her anymore and did my best to promote her independence. I knew school wasn't going as well as we both wanted, but I tried consoling her and tried giving her strategies to make it through the high school years.

In her four years of high school, I went to her yearly IEP meetings, parent/teacher conferences, and maybe made a phone call or two. I didn't want to be "that" mom that was always bugging teachers and constantly asking them for more. I have known a lot of teachers over the years and can't imagine how challenging it might be to try to make every parent and child happy. I didn't want to be the complainer. I regret this time in Lindsey's education.

When Lindsey posted her *Facebook* message about how unhappy she was, my phone began ringing. Besides family and friends calling me, her elementary teachers called me. I couldn't ignore it anymore. Lindsey had just given a speech about autism at an elementary school in Wisconsin. The speech was about her positive elementary years and being included. It also talked about her high school years of not having classmates that understood her or wanted to be with her. I printed off a copy of it and the *Facebook* post. Four years of frustration was built up inside of me when I called her high school to request a meeting with the principal. I insisted the meeting take place immediately. I told them I would be at school in fifteen minutes. Shaking, I held the papers in my hand as I walked through the high school doors. I begged the principal, "Please read these." As he read them, all he could say was, "I am so sorry." He was next to speechless. He told me that he wished he could change things for Lindsey, but there were only four weeks left of school.

Even if things weren't going to change, I felt good when I left the high school building. I had heard year after year that the school was going to try to help Lindsey with friendships. However, they would comment, "We can't make the kids be her friend." I was relieved that I had the courage to share my feelings. Within a couple of hours, I received a phone call from the principal about the prom proposal that he was trying to make happen. He bought the prom tickets, he lent her date a tie that would match her dress, and did whatever he could to make it a happy experience for her. I was torn up inside. What if I had approached him sooner? At the same time, I was grateful.

As Lindsey's previous chapter shows so well, she had an amazing prom. As happy as I felt about it, I still worried about it. I didn't want her getting picked on, and I didn't want her date getting picked on. I called his parents. They reassured me that he really wanted to take Lindsey to prom. He told them that he didn't feel like he **had** to or felt forced to take her. It put me at ease so that we could all enjoy the day. Her date did something for Lindsey beyond any words I could ever express. Lindsey's joyous expression during the grand march that night is something I will always cherish. What a wonderful young man to step up and selflessly give her this memory.

Chapter Forty-Two

"I would say that college was worth it."

By Lindsey Moreland

In the last week of August 2012, I started going to college. I went to a technical college for general classes. I was surprised that I had low placement test scores since I had graduated with honors in high school. Because of my low test scores, I had to take pre-college courses. It was embarrassing and humiliating. I felt like the teacher was arrogant and a "know-it-all" teacher and here she was teaching in a classroom for students with learning differences. She thought I was stupid because I think and learn differently. She didn't understand autism. One time she made me teary because she had a poor attitude, and it was causing me anxiety. Other than that, I did well in my courses. In fact, on April 2013, I received a scholarship from this same technical college.

I also went to a Wisconsin university to study Spanish. Intermediate Spanish class was actually fun and easy for me to learn. I was one of the top students in this class. The professor was funny, but also sometimes made me a bit nervous because he mentioned that not all students did well on their tests, except me! I enjoyed this class. Spring semester, I was a top student again. I appreciated that he expressed that he was pleased with how hard I was working. He asked me to be part of the *Spanish Professions of Association.*

In 2013, college started to get stressful. I had a different professor in Spanish who completely made me anxious and terrified. I felt her attitude was horrible and she was unkind. If someone in the class answered wrong, she would get mad and say, "You're doing it wrong!" I was not the only one who felt uncomfortable and terrified. I rarely participated in her class because I was afraid of answering the questions wrong, because I knew she would go ballistic, and then I would be embarrassed.

Fall semester in 2014, I was overloaded with work, and it was complete hell for me. I had way too many homework assignments to get done at the same time. I had more than one test to take in the same week. I had four classes, two at CVTC and two Spanish classes at UWRF. I was excited to be in Spanish Trades for Professions class and have the professor who I had before, but things went wrong. With all the hard work, I felt overwhelmed with disappointment when I got a "C" on one test. The nice professor said that I didn't do well. He also asked me, "What happened?" I was embarrassed and humiliated. Did he say that because he cared for me so much that he was concerned? Or, did he say that because he was frustrated? I was working so hard studying all the time, again had no time to socialize because of my anxiety.

During this semester, I had Spanish Literature class with the professor who terrified me. I got a passing average grade on my quiz, and she said to the class that they didn't do well. She even made a terrible joke that if we didn't do well again, we might as well jump off the bridge. The students were laughing, but I wasn't because suicidal jokes were not appropriate.

Another challenging part of that semester was that I had to walk from the technical college to the university back and forth several times a day. I walked extremely fast to get there on time due to my phobia of being late. I felt even more exhausted. It was the last semester of going to the technical college because I planned to be a full-time student at the university. Since this was all difficult, I knew going to one location would help me. Even when I was on Christmas break, I couldn't relax and was sick to my stomach. The spring semester was better than the previous semester. I got the professor with the good sense of humor, and I was his top student in Spanish Professions of Writing. The only negative part was that on a Monday in February, I fell on the ice and broke my shoulder bone. According to the doctor's orders, I had to stay home for a couple a days. It made me anxious because I dislike missing days of classes. I did eventually send email to my professors about my incident, and they were completely nice and understandable.

In the summer of 2015, I decided to declare an Elementary Education major with a minor in Spanish because I love working with and teaching children.

In the fall semester of 2015, I thought that it was going okay. I was still stressed with the overload of assignments and tests, though. Again, I had the professor who terrified me. She was a bit better with her attitude, but one time, she was completely unhappy about how we did on our midterm. She mentioned that, "We weren't working hard enough, and this isn't high school!" First of all, I was working hard enough. Second, why have I hardly socialized when I was busy with my studies every day. Third, there are other classes I have to worry about too. No one is perfect for goodness sake! In fact, I got a "B+" on that midterm, which was close to an "A-." She almost had me in tears. The next day, I felt sick to my stomach because I was afraid of what the professor would say or do next. I was one of her top students in that class. During finals week one day, I spent ten hours studying. After I did well with this semester, I didn't get sick, but I overslept a lot due to my stress level.

Spring semester of 2016 was better than I expected. In Advanced Spanish class, I had the newest and nicest professor who had a similar personality to my high school Spanish teacher. I was still independent with my studies. I had classes that kept me extremely busy. I hardly had the time to socialize. I've been an introvert my entire life, and this was frustrating to me. Again, during finals week, I studied around ten hours per day. That semester, I got straight A's and made it on the Dean's list.

Part of the summer of 2016 was stressful because part of Elementary Education is taking the *Praxis* exams. After finishing the semester, I was exhausted, and I overslept. I spent way too much time studying again. One evening I was completely frustrated that college was causing me stress and anxiety that my Mom thought it would be best for me to take a break.

I don't like to talk about this, but people often ask me about my college years and why I didn't finish my degree. For health reasons, I decided it was best for me to relook at a career that I felt would suit me better. I feel great success in what I have already accomplished. No amount of college is a waste of time or money. During college, I had a crazy obsession over studying that caused me social anxiety and made me feel sick often. With my obsession of studying, I was hardly eating, even though I didn't try to lose weight. Even when I was on a seasonal break I was feeling sick and anxious about college. Even though professors probably didn't expect everyone to be a 4.0 student, I felt I needed to be. My G.P.A. was 3.75, which my mom tells me how proud she is of me, and she realized how hard it really was on me. At first I didn't want to go to college because studying caused anxiety. I didn't want to deal with more sadness. I felt bad that I couldn't socialize. For example, I did not go to my sister's dance class due to my fear. My parents thought college would be different than high school. I wanted to please them, so I went. At the time I was not happy about this, but my parents didn't realize it. There are positive memories I have of college. In the summer of 2014, I traveled to Mexico, and in the fall semester of 2014, I was Vice President for Spanish Professions of Association. Because of my college, I decided to become a paraprofessional.

My family and friends are very happy for my decision. They completely understand and accept my life choices. From 2016-2017, I volunteered at 2 elementary school districts, 40 hours a week. My aunt, who is a teacher, put together a plan to help me become employed. My job duties were helping to correct papers, organizing classroom materials, translating documents, working with Spanish-speaking students, and being involved with reading groups. I loved helping the teachers and the students. It's one of the reasons why I decided I want to become a paraprofessional. I also have a dream to become a motivational speaker and to be an activist against bullying.

Chapter Forty-Three

"It will get better...or will it?"

By Brittany Moreland, Lindsey's sister

Lindsey and I had a great relationship growing up and still do today. I feel like I can relate to her and empathize with her when she talks about being bullied, ignored, and left out. It seems like most people I talk to have a story about being bullied, picked on, or left out. Why does it continue? Grown-ups will tell you, "It will get better...you just have to get through it." I often hear people say that it stops when you get out of school, but it doesn't always. They also say that everyone goes through it. I have a hard time believing that everyone goes through the amount of bullying Lindsey and I endured.

When Lindsey and I were in elementary, middle, and high school, bus rides and the lunchroom were the worst. I would add physical education class to that list as well. Whether the behaviors of others were considered mean, rude, or bullying, they were extremely hurtful. Each day, I would ask multiple kids if I could sit with them on the bus. Some would move their backpack to save the space for someone else. Sometimes they would just say, "No." Other times, they would roll their eyes. Even kids who I thought were my friends would say, "No." Lindsey had such a hard time with it that eventually the bus driver gave her a reserved seat in the front which ended up getting her picked on even more.

Mean behavior from students included being ditched on the playground. Games would be made up to exclude others. When kids were picking teams, I was often last or second to last. While other kids might have similar experiences, I had the extra layer of having a seizure disorder. Kids said I was lucky to have it because I could get notes that would excuse me from activities. I could also have extra time on tests. I was able to get extra help from the teachers. I was able to leave class early to get to the next class because I was having trouble telling time and moved slower due to my medications. Students picked on me for these differences. How could they think that I was lucky? I will never forget the time that a student acted out a seizure in an improvisational play, and everyone laughed. I also remember science class where the joke of the class was learning about seizures and having to act them out. If you have never had a seizure, you do not understand the severity of the experience. Imagine your brain starts to get foggy. You feel paralyzed and exhausted. Your body falls to the floor, and you begin shaking uncontrollably. Trying to breathe, your airway feels clogged, and you begin to drool. While this is happening, you see people around you freaking out, and you can't tell them how to help you. Confused, you wonder when it will end. It may only last a couple of minutes, but it feels like forever. Lying on your side, you feel helpless, as you wait for it to be over. Because I have had two Grand Mal seizures, any minor seizure activity made me nervous, worried, and anxious.

I hated changing in front of others in gym class, so I would change in the bathroom. Girls would comment and pick on me for this. They called it stupid and laughed at me. Being picked on so much, I became a loner. I became shy and super sad. I wore my emotions on my sleeve, and it was hard not to cry. When I cried, I would get picked on for that, so I tried laughing when the other kids laughed. Basically, I was just trying to survive. In high school, I would have to go to the nurse to take naps because I was shaking so much. One student said I was lucky and wished he could take naps at school. I couldn't believe he really felt that way. I cried on the bed in the nurse's office and wanted to make a change.

When the summer of 2009 came, I was determined to make that change. My seizures decreased and I was able to go off of medication. My depression continued to skyrocket to the point where my mom had to rip the covers off of me to get me out of bed. That summer I had a lot of intense therapy. One of my dreams growing up was to go skydiving. Thinking about all that I had been through, I decided skydiving would be a way to emotionally start fresh. It would symbolize a new me. Jumping out of that airplane was my way of showing myself that I had the courage to do anything and accomplish my goals if I set my mind to it.

My senior year was much better. I reached out to a couple girls that I thought would be my friends. Several turned me down because they thought I was still the "sick kid." Maybe they didn't want to ruin their reputation. I could only speculate. Two girls accepted my request to be their friend. We went to football games and even prom. I now had partners in class that actually wanted to be my partner. Sadly, Lindsey never was able to make a friend in high school.

Why talk about all this bullying and depression? Why bring up all of the painful memories especially when others say they have been through hard times too? I am sharing it because it is not only a part of the story, it is a way to make a difference for others. I have been asked, "What can people do so that kids change the way they treat each other?" "What can educators and parents do to help?" I have come up with a few things that I think would have helped Lindsey and me.

- Students: If a child is shy or quiet, try to talk to them. If they don't respond, it doesn't mean they don't want you to try again. Keep trying. Shy kids and kids with differences want friends. Talking to them will help them gain the social skills they need to make friends.

- Students: If you see someone getting picked on or ignored, step up and talk to them.
- Students: Smile and say hello to everyone. Acknowledge their presence.
- Students: If you don't have something nice to say, don't say anything at all. Quiet kids and kids with special needs can hear you. They are listening, and they have feelings just like you.
- Students: Ask your teachers what to do if you don't know how to talk or interact with someone who has differences or a medical condition.
- Educators: Educate students about different special needs. Don't stop educating them or think that one time is enough. A refresher lesson needs to happen often. Scenarios where children imagine living a day in the life of a special needs child could help children better understand that a child is not "weird" or "strange."
- Educators: Organize friendship groups in elementary, middle, **and** high school. Reach out to kids that may want to help or may also need a friend.

- Educators: Assign partners instead of having students pick. Think about how you are assigning them.
- Educators: Send out a survey to your families asking families if they would be willing to make connections with families who have special needs children.
- Educators: Give incentives to students who reach out and befriend others who need a friend.
- Parents: Encourage your child to invite students with a special need or disability for a play date.
- Parents: Listen and encourage your child to try things even if you feel like it might not work out for your child.
- Parents: Talk to your child with special-needs, and explain why you are making certain decisions. For example, my dad never told me that he decided to get a family dog to help me with my seizures and depression. I wish he would have been more open.

Changes need to be made so that all children feel included, supported, and wanted. I can't change what happened to Lindsey or me. I also don't want to dwell on the past. However, the experiences of your younger years are a part of life and can make or break you. Luckily, I am not broken, but it has given me a purpose to help others have a better life.

Chapter Forty-Four

"Vulnerable Adult"

By Lauri Moreland, Lindsey's mom

After Lindsey graduated high school with honors, we still had a lot of work ahead of us to get her into college. In high school, Lindsey had anxiety about taking college preparatory classes. She also stated that she did not want to go to college. When she changed her mind, it was too late for her to be able to complete all of those classes. Lindsey took the ACT (American College Testing) exam and scored 15 which was significantly below the cut score to be accepted at a university. A university in Wisconsin suggested she take pre-college courses at a technical college. She could still take Spanish classes at the university. Because she tested out of a year of Spanish through their placement test, they offered her the opportunity to attend college and be a full time student. We declined because we thought that it would be better for her to start out at a smaller school. At the technical college, she took a placement test which reported her academic functioning level.

Although she didn't love it there, she was successful. Interacting with staff was sometimes challenging for her. The online classes were especially difficult because Lindsey does best when she has a visual right in front of her along with a teacher. According to Lindsey, most of the students were kind. They would say, "Hello," and "How are you?" That was the extent of it. She didn't spend time with them outside of school.

In the fall semester of 2014, Lindsey came home and said that she had met a friend. I was surprised and hopeful. I was even more surprised when she said the friend was a boy. She told me that she was going to meet him on a Sunday at a coffee shop downtown. I began asking questions about the young man. She told me which class she had with him, and according to her he was around her same age. A part of me was excited for this chance at friendship. However, I was also concerned due to her limited experience with friends. All other friendship experiences were either paid or supervised. I had other plans for the day, and I wouldn't be around in case she needed me. Brittany was running a 5K race an hour way, and I was going to drive her there to cheer her on. Todd might have been available, but Lindsey would call me when she needed help with most things.

Lindsey was living in an apartment with her sister and a roommate in town. She also had a room at our house where she could stay. We were working on helping her become more independent. So, on a cold, October, Sunday, Lindsey walked down to the local coffee shop. Brittany and I went to the race. During the race, I got a frantic phone call from Lindsey. Lindsey was crying and said, "I have been standing outside the coffee shop freezing for an hour....and he hasn't showed up!" He had told her that they would meet outside the coffee shop-not inside, and of course Lindsey followed that direction regardless of the frigid temperature. I felt terrible that I was not there for her to console her and give her a ride home. Lindsey was extremely upset ranting about mean people, all of the studying time she was missing out on, and the stress of the entire experience. I let her know that I would be there as soon as possible. After the race, Brittany and I picked her up at her apartment, and I brought her home. Immediately, I gave her deep pressure therapy and really tight hugs. I did my best to help her calm down and make her feel better.

Asking more questions about this man, I became concerned. Lindsey knew his full name, so I did some research on the internet. Shocked, I found that he had an extensive criminal record including robbery. He was 33 years old (13 years older than Lindsey)! I went from being frustrated with this man to being relieved that he didn't actually show up. Lindsey became more upset.

"I'm sorry," she cried. She felt stupid and thought she should know better. She had been tricked by someone she thought was being nice to her and wanted to get to know her.

Immediately, I called the police department. I called the non-emergency number and had a conversation with an officer about what we should do about this situation. I explained that Lindsey had autism and that I felt that she was a vulnerable adult. I knew that there wasn't any legal action required, but I wanted to protect Lindsey from a possible encounter with this man in the future. The man had been arrested multiple times for various things which was a huge concern for all of us. Of course people change, but it didn't make me feel any better. Upon the officer's suggestions, I called the technical college. They were aware of his past, and reported that he was rehabilitating. Although they couldn't do anything because of his past, they would "keep an eye" on the situation.

Lindsey returned to school, but did not engage in communication with him. He continued to text her even though she wouldn't return his texts. He tried for a few weeks and even sent her a "Happy Thanksgiving" text. Eventually it stopped. As a parent of an adult with autism, this is a constant fear. Lindsey has learned that she can and should talk to us about any situation that does or doesn't feel right to her.

One other time when she was walking to her next class at the university, a male approached her and asked her if the town had an adult video store. Lindsey replied that she didn't know and kept on walking. He pulled out his phone and tried showing her a pornographic video. She did the right thing. She kept walking, didn't look at him, and went to the nearest building. He left her alone. Months passed. Lindsey decided to go to the movie alone. She had gotten movie tickets from her great grandma and wanted to honor her passing the day after her death by going to the movies. As she was standing in line, this same man approached her again. He asked the same questions and tried to show her the video. Again, Lindsey did the right thing by ignoring him. She also called me. It was another time that "nothing" was actually done to her, but it was still scary. Later, we read an article in the paper about the man. He was doing the same thing to other women around town. Bravely, Lindsey called the police department and told them her experience. Brittany and I also talked to the police. I requested that Lindsey not have to testify if they already had enough women to make their criminal case against him. Fortunately or unfortunately, they did.

These incidents remind me how important it is to stay involved in Lindsey's life no matter what age. I will always want to protect her and work through unexpected and unwanted experiences that she may encounter. As a parent of an adult with autism, it is important to ask questions often and investigate individuals who are involved in their life.

This also means being involved in helping your adult child get employed. A lot of kids and adults that have autism can and want to work. How does a family and our society aid this? School had to be modified, and work will have to be modified. Employers need to get involved by learning about their employee's abilities. They can help by tailoring work for them. If given the chance, an adult with autism could be a huge asset for a company. In fact, they will probably be one of your best employees. The community needs to step up and get involved, too. Having a job often leads to making friends with coworkers. Adults with autism want friends.

People who have autism often have social anxiety regardless of how smart they are or how different they seem. I have lost sleep over my wonders and Lindsey's future as a vulnerable adult along with all of the other vulnerable adults in our society. What will happen to these adults if we don't find a way to get them employed? Lindsey is currently looking for a job. This has not been easy. Above all, it has been extremely stressful. She has been on 5 interviews. She has felt great after the interviews and is always positive and hopeful. Independently, she has applied for these jobs and set up the interviews. She has the qualifications and schooling to get hired. We consider this a success. However, she feels defeated when she gets the call or the e-mail that someone was chosen over her. It is hard not to call the employer and question why they won't give her a chance. She is a visual learner. Maybe if she had a way to show her skills versus verbally explain them, she would convince an employer that she is a good candidate to get the job. She will need a patient employer in a day and age where there isn't always patience. She will need help with social situations in the workplace. She communicates in different ways. She's a concrete thinker. Her senses are different than mine. Lindsey has many successes, but there are still so many challenges. Many of these challenges the outside world cannot see or understand that it does not make her less capable of working. One of these is auditory delay. However, once she understands what is being asked of her, she follows through with impeccable detail and completion. Recently, we have reached out to DVR (Division of Vocational Rehabilitation) to assist us in helping Lindsey become employed. Lindsey is continuing to try and get a job on her own while she waits for DVR's involvement. For qualifying individuals, this program includes multiple components. This may include, but is not limited to, finding a job, planning your career, getting skills and necessary education for the job, and job coaching.

Getting a job is at the top of her priority list right now, and just think about how positive this will be for her self-esteem once she is hired.

Chapter Forty-Five

"I'll be there for you."

By Brittany Moreland, Lindsey's sister

While school was a challenge, I was fortunate that our family was able to share many good times together. We traveled to *Disney World* twice. One summer, we vacationed in California. That was the trip Lindsey bought a trophy for herself titled, "Person of the Year." Every Christmas Eve, we went to the *Mall of America* which was a special treat because our mom hated driving in busy traffic. Dad would wait for hours as we tried on clothes. We spent a lot of time on the lake fishing, swimming, and paddle boating. Lindsey loved creating comedy shows. I would videotape her and she would tell me when I could laugh. As a family, we watched the shows after dinner. The love from my family didn't stop there. My extended family which included my mom's parents, aunts, uncles, and cousins shared many great memories, too. They welcomed my differences and didn't judge me for them. I always felt included. We got together often. We loved jamming in the music room with grandpa, playing softball, football, and kickball, making crafts with grandma, and playing intense card games. These are my best childhood memories.

As an adult with a healthier mindset, I feel closer to my family than I ever have. I have learned that I need to respectfully share my feelings and make arrangements to hang out with them more instead of holding onto my feelings or shutting them out. We enjoy walks together, play games, and watch movies. In my senior year of high school, I joined a dance studio and developed a passion for all types of dancing and went on to become a dance instructor a few years later. I convinced my dad to join me for a father/daughter dance recital in 2010. This wasn't something I thought my dad would ever want to do, but he did it just for me knowing how important dance was in my life. The bear hunting trip to Canada with my dad in the summer of 2016 was a great bonding experience. Since then, I feel even closer to him. My mom supported me modeling in Chicago. Even though she was recovering from influenza and needed to take off a whole week of work, she was determined to be there for me. One of my favorite memories with my mom is dancing together to my uncle's band. We were the first ones on the dance floor, and the last ones to leave the dance floor.

I know this hasn't been easy on my parents. No one in my family asked to go through depression, autism, and seizures. Yet, this was the hand we were dealt, and my parents learned to play with the cards they were given. I know I am blessed that our family has somehow stuck it out together. Research shows high rates of divorce, and family animosity with families that deal with special needs. There are things we are going to disagree on. There are happy memories and sad memories, just like any other family. I can't tell you how lucky I am to have them both. I am also blessed by the amazing friends I have in my life. They are kind, caring, and amazing to my sister. I lost a lot of friends because of my epilepsy and depression in the past. When I was in college I broke down to a friend. I was worried she wouldn't want to be my friend anymore because that is what happened in the past. She told me, "I'm still going to be your friend...just because you cry, share a bad day, or are going through a hard time doesn't mean you're going to lose this friendship over that." That was the best thing I had heard and appreciated it so much. I still get anxiety sharing sad things to others because there's a little fear that they might leave, but I know now that your true friends will stay with you through the good and the bad times.

Last month, I gave a speech at St. Catherine's University in Minnesota with my mom and sister about how autism impacted our lives and continues to impact it. A student asked me a question that really made me feel good about how far our family has come throughout the years. She commented on how hard our lives had been and wondered about our future. She asked, "What do you enjoy in life now that autism is not the number one factor?" I told her that autism is still a part of our life and will be forever. We still make decisions as a result of it, but we can do so many more things than I ever imagined we would be able to do. It is the simple things in life that others take for granted and I am truly grateful.

I can hug my sister. I can do her hair. We can have conversations and she understands what I am saying. We love dancing together. We can even go to a concert where there are lots of people in small spaces and the noise is deafening. We can cook together and go to the movie theater. Believe it or not, we don't even have to watch the same movie over and over. Lindsey used to hate going shopping, especially for clothes. At the mall, she rarely entered the store, but she was polite about it-with a, "No thank you." Now, we can shop until we drop. We talk about our futures and getting married. Just a couple weeks ago, Lindsey's boyfriend, my boyfriend, and my parents enjoyed a fun evening together celebrating my mom's birthday. We are best friends! When she is sad, I am sad. When she is happy, I am happy.

I worry a lot less about Lindsey now because she is doing so well. A situation that happened recently reminds me that I don't need to be as protective as I have been in the past. She has a mind of her own and isn't afraid to share her thoughts with me. I have always tried to include

Lindsey when I hang out with friends and have let her crash many of my dates. When Lindsey started dating her boyfriend this past year, I asked if I could meet him and crash her date. First, she made an excuse saying that she had to check their schedules. I kept bugging her about it and even texted him. He replied that I could hang out with them. Lindsey said, "To be honest Brittany....I want it to be just Zach and me time." She continued, "There have been many times that I have not come on your dates. I feel bad, but I just want it to be the two of us, not you." I was offended and sad. My parents had already met him. This was a lot different than what I was used to. If Lindsey didn't like a guy I was dating, he never met my parents. Her approval was number one for me. I got a call from my mom later that day explaining that Lindsey was upset. She told my mom, "You and dad have your time. Brittany and her boyfriend have her time. I have never had this, and it's my turn now!" The next morning after I apologized, Lindsey sent me a text saying, "It's ok. Now we are even." I think it's great that Lindsey and I can talk and laugh about this now. The even better thing is that my mom doesn't have to be involved in helping Lindsey communicate with me.

Our journey continues with both good times and bad. With the experiences I have gone through, I have learned to have strength, kindness, courage, and love. I have learned not to judge others because you don't know another person's story. It could be worse than yours, it could be similar or it could be better. Being a part of my sister's story has been a crazy rollercoaster ride, but I wouldn't choose to go on any other ride.

As we look ahead to our future, we love talking about weddings and what our future holds. One time we even made a *PowerPoint* of our wedding dreams. We deleted it immediately when my mom joked, "Now you just need to find a guy and this could scare a guy away." Reluctantly, Lindsey has allowed me to share that she has a secret *Pinterest* wedding board. Our future is bright, but we will take it one day at a time.

Chapter Forty-Six

"Thanks for the memories."

By Ida Feyereisen, Lindsey's Grandma

Lindsey is fortunate to have been born to a loving family who has supported her throughout the years and continues to support her. As the girls were growing up, Todd was there to spend time with them and see to it that they had everything a therapist would suggest or that he himself felt would help to make both of them happy.

When Lindsey was going to college, she was living with Brittany in an apartment near campus. Brittany was always there for her sister by letting her parents know when she saw Lindsey was having an issue with food, school, homework, or just life in general.

Brittany has worked through so many challenges. The doctors tell Brittany that some of her seizure activity is caused by stress. She is learning how to reduce the stress in her life. She has a job using her cosmetology degree in the warehouse and office of a company that sells hair products to cosmetologists. Since she also enjoys using the products her company sells, she is able to promote these products. Lots of friends and family members have benefited from her hair coloring and styling talent. She has had her work featured in *Wisconsin Bride* magazine. She has also been a hair model for several famous stylists at large hair shows in the Midwest. I'm proud of her. She has come so far.

There was no one who was a better advocate for her children than Lauri. She has dealt with the everyday issues and challenges that come with raising a child with autism and the special needs of a sibling of that child.

When the girls were very young, I was working part time and felt bad that I couldn't be more helpful. Lauri and I talked on the phone at least once or twice each day. I knew she was hurting, and I could do nothing to change that. All I could do was encourage her to hang in there and never give up, and she never did.

I'll never forget the day when Lindsey was young, and they were visiting us. It was still typical for Lindsey to have what most of us would call a tantrum when she wasn't able to communicate her needs. The kicking, screaming, and head banging put her in a situation where she might hurt herself. They had already learned that firm pressure worked better for Lindsey than a light touch. I could hardly watch as Lauri struggled to pick her up, and literally used all of her strength to restrain her and put her in a tight hold. Eventually, Lindsey could resist no longer and she melted briefly in Lauri's arms. Lauri asked her if she wanted a drink of milk, and she jumped up and ran to the refrigerator as if this hadn't even happened.

I see the challenges Lauri faces change gradually as the girls grow older, but they never go away. Lauri has always been there, and will always be there to deal with whatever situations arise. We know it's not always going to be easy, but she will never give up.

Although Brittany and Lindsey had so many, negative experiences during their childhood, I'm happy to hear that both of the girls have great memories from the times they spent here at our home with their cousins. The time we've spent with our grandchildren have given Steve, Lindsey's grandpa, and me the best memories. We were blessed to have 15 wonderful grandchildren in a period of 10 years, and that they all grew up living close enough to us that we could be a part of their growing up years. Sadly, the only exception was baby Nicholas who died of SIDS (Sudden Infant Death Syndrome) at only 6 weeks of age. We still count him, because we still have him. We just can't hug him.

All of our grandkids have super parents that were nice enough to let us babysit, and spend time with the kids here at our house. They enjoyed many indoor and outdoor activities together, including climbing the big climbing tree and reminiscing around the campfire.

The sandbox occupied several grandkids at a time for hours at a time. Lindsey played there too, but she enjoyed it most if she was alone or just with Brittany. It would be a great place to be creative with a few old trucks, tractors and dozers.

We learned that there was no point in forcing a child with autism to squeeze into the group of 14 squirming kids to get their picture taken. In one of these outdoor pictures Lindsey can be seen sitting on the trike. She seemed to feel safe hanging on to something while the others sat in the grass. Another time when all the rest of the kids were on the wagon Grandpa Steve was pulling with his lawn tractor, Lindsey was on his lap. That crowd was too much for her, but we learned how to get great pictures that included her.

All the grandkids started out playing and singing with Grandpa Steve in his music room from very little on. They first used kazoos, castanets, and little cordless microphones I made for our own kids years ago. I crocheted them out of blue yarn and stuffed them with batting. We still have those and now our great grandchildren are using them. Eventually they advanced to real instruments including a full drum set. The room is small and Lindsey seems to be uncomfortable in there with a group of kids, although she had played her guitar in there with Grandpa in the past. It's just one of those things she doesn't enjoy right now, but maybe someday she will try it again.

Lindsey and I have enjoyed some projects over the years, just like I have with the other grandkids. She made cookies with me a few times before we realized she was sensitive to gluten. She came and sewed a little, long shoulder strap purse in just one day.

Brittany remembers the time she asked me to help her make a wedding cake for a 4-H foods project for the county fair. She felt so defeated when I told her I had never made one and knew the challenge was way too much for a beginner. I suggested we make decorated, rolled out cookies instead. She reluctantly agreed and found out even that was a challenge. Once I helped her make a pillow that I thought was a unique, but simple project. However, sewing on 6 large buttons became a challenge. She sure learned to sew on buttons and we can laugh about that now.

Once when I was playing Yahtzee with a few of the grandkids, Lindsey got so impatient with the rest of us when we had to count the spots on the dice. She could take one look at the five dice and give us a quick total. It bothered her so that she actually had to walk away from the game. However, we all laughed (including her) when she kept peeking around the corner telling us the totals.

When the grandkids were little and I was still working part time from home, I was able to have some of them part time or full time for a while when their mothers worked. We often spent time coloring or drawing at the kitchen table. Some remember Grandpa drawing them tractors. He was definitely the better artist. We kept putting the pictures up on the refrigerator until I had to take some down to make room for more. I was getting a big collection of pictures. I didn't want to throw them away but where would I put them? I bought a stack of spiral notebooks and gave one to each child. They each put their names on the cover, and each time they came they were to draw one nice picture and put their name and date on the picture. This way I'd be able to save them all and see the progress they were making. When their book got full, they got a new one. One day I noticed Brittany was scribbling on every page of her book. I was pretty upset about it, because I knew she could draw so nice and she wasn't following the rules. Recently, Brittany, Lindsey, their Aunt Nancy and Cousin Stephanie came to visit us. We talked about those books. They got them out to look at and ended up drawing, dating, and signing another page. Brittany laughed about her scribbling incident and said Jake had filled his book and got a new one and she wanted a new one too. It worked. I bring all of this up because drawing back then was not something Lindsey spent a lot of time doing at our house. Maybe there were too many kids around the table.

By now of course you know that Lindsey is a pencil artist. She has become so much more social now as an adult and enjoys time with her parents, her boyfriend and her sister. Drawing is something she can do on her alone time. I love all of her drawings, but I think her animals are so special. She gives each animal a personality, especially our special 9 year old cocker/springer, Molly.

I have learned that every child with autism is different. Perhaps there is another child somewhere that is just like Lindsey, with the same talents, the same feelings, the same wants out of life, but I doubt it. I believe she is one of a kind and she has taught me to never judge anyone. God has blessed her with parents and a sister who have always been and always will be a wonderful part of her life. She is also blessed to have her very special Aunt Linda who has spent countless hours these last few years mentoring her, encouraging her, and helping write her story. Yes, "They will all have her back," and she will have theirs.

Chapter Forty-Seven

"Fortunately"

By Lauri Moreland, Lindsey's mom

Never in my dreams could I have imagined that at 23 years old, Lindsey would have a bright future. I am proud to say today that I truly believe she does. Of course she will have hard times and hard days with challenges along the way. When we share our story at schools, conferences, and universities, the questions most frequently asked are "What do you think made the biggest change?" "What helped the most?" and "What do you see for your future?"

In my opinion, there isn't just one thing that made the biggest change. I can't say for sure what really worked. We were doing everything at the same time. Many factors contributed to Lindsey's success story. First, when she was diagnosed with autism, I read everything I could about it. I spent hours and days finding out as much information about a word I had never heard. Although what I read did not give me much hope, I was determined. Twenty-two years ago, the outlook for a child with autism seemed to be a predictable future and not a good one. I wasn't going to sit around and believe in that. Lindsey started therapy at 15 months. This was speech therapy and included blowing bubbles, water play, and taking turns. After her official diagnosis at 28 months, early intervention was recommended. I was completely on board. I did not hesitate to even think that she could improve without help. Occupational therapy, physical therapy, and sensory integration were added the following week. Luckily, our private insurance covered these therapies. We were blessed when the special education center she was going to, decided to forgive our copayments.

Lindsey's favorite and most helpful experiences through her therapies were water play, pillow piles, wrapping her in blankets, swinging, the ball pit, the trampoline, a weighted vest, a quiet environment when needed, and playing in shaving cream. Brushing her skin with a surgical brush was effective for desensitizing her skin even though she didn't like it. Auditory training was added at 3 years old. I wanted to believe that it would calm her down and help lessen the tantrums. It claimed it would also improve her ability to focus. We used sign language and Mayer Johnson symbols until she became verbal. Lindsey had a favorite shirt called her "Blue, Butterfly Shirt." We used it as a tool to reinforce positive behavior and eating. When she was hospitalized, it was the only thing that worked in getting her to eat. We relied on social stories to help explain her day and any other upcoming situations. Her gluten free diet seemed to calm her and alleviate her stomach issues. Fortunately, Lindsey's behavior and communication continued to improve throughout her years of therapy. Periodically, she would regress, but then it would be followed with a monumental gain.

There were so many things that I did for Lindsey to help her, but there were also things that I did to help survive the day to day life of being a parent of a child with autism. I made sure our life was as organized as possible and followed a routine that she could understand. I allowed her to stay in her pajamas all day if that is what she wanted. I challenged her on days when I felt I was up for it. For example, if I felt emotionally strong on a particular day, I would drive a different route to my parents' house with the goal of helping Lindsey accept change. I could handle her screaming and kicking the back seat of the car on certain days. I used movies to ease the challenging times such as haircuts, rest time, and as a reward for eating. When others stared at us or looked at me in a judging way, I did my best to smile and not give them my opinion about our situation. I relied on my family and we stayed busy.

With regards to our future, we are all positive. We look forward to spending time together as a family. When Brittany told an audience at one of our speaking engagements this year, that we were a happy family who enjoyed simple things and didn't take anything for granted, I was especially proud. It was an "ah ha" moment that our family was now surviving and thriving.

Chapter Forty-Eight

"Our Marriage is a Contract for Life"

By Todd Moreland, Lindsey's dad

Lauri and I are sitting here today talking about the memories we have shared since we met over 30 years ago. No one could have prepared the two of us for the life we would live with autism and epilepsy. We had never even heard the word autism and knew very little about epilepsy. Lauri always wanted to talk about it. I was dealing with it in a much different way than Lauri. I don't feel like I was avoiding it. I just couldn't talk about it. I suppose I was in denial. I didn't want to accept the fact that there could be anything wrong with Lindsey, and I couldn't believe it, when Brittany started having seizures.

We wanted to be like most married couples, but we really weren't. It wasn't possible to even think about going out to dinner or to a movie. It wouldn't have been enjoyable. Lauri couldn't stop thinking about autism, and we couldn't call just anyone, including a teenage neighbor girl to babysit.

Lauri just wanted to "fix" Lindsey and "cure" her of autism. When Lindsey was between 3 and 4 years old, Lauri was so exhausted from dealing with the tantrums. She told me that she pleaded with the doctor, and convinced him, to prescribe medication for Lindsey, even though he said it wasn't going to cure her autism. My response was "absolutely not, we are not medicating her" and we never did. Lauri and I both understand now and recognize that some people with autism benefit greatly from medication depending on their situation. At the time, it sounded to me like the doctor thought pills would do nothing-so what was the point? Lauri said that I could stay home and she would go to work, but she didn't go to work, so I continued to work. I was the one who could work days 40 to 60 hours a week and be home in the evenings to spend time with her and the girls. My responsibilities at home also included plowing the snow, mowing the grass, doing any needed home & vehicle repairs, and helping with some of the grocery shopping and preparing some meals. It wasn't like we sat down and pointed out who would do what; it just worked out that way.

Lauri admits that she didn't even have the strength to start the lawn mower, shovel snow, or run the snow blower. However, we both knew that Lauri was much better at handling the ongoing day to day struggles with the girls at home and at school. She handled all the meetings, phone calls, autism research, doctor & therapy appointments, and our household finances, along with all the needs of running a normal household. In the evenings I often took the girls shopping, to the park, and to Burger

King to get Lindsey chicken nuggets. That is all she would eat at the time.

When Lauri started working 3 evenings a week at the barber shop, I took the girls to the river to feed the ducks, and when I got the boat, I took them out on the lake. This gave Lauri the opportunity to keep up her cosmetology license and I knew she needed this time away. It's like whatever works, works. We didn't really fight. If Lauri wanted something, I went along with it. If I wanted something, she went along with it too. We didn't argue about money and that helped. The stress in our relationship was always the kids.

As we sit and talk about these memories, Lauri talks about being the nagger, the complainer, and the crier. On hard days I was the one that just let it blow over. I waited it out. I figured Lindsey's tantrums would just go away. When Brittany started having seizures, there were times when she needed to be picked up at school 3 or 4 times a week. I could get off work to get her, but Lauri couldn't. I took her to a lot of doctor appointments. Lauri can't help but think that she got stuck with a lot of the crap, and I guess she did. Lauri wished the girls would have gone to me with more of their problems. She was the one who had to break Brittany's heart and be honest with her when she had so many big hopes and dreams. Sadly, at that time, I was dealing more with their physical needs and not with their feelings and emotions. My way of dealing with it was to give them good experiences.

We are able to laugh and joke that the many moves we made and the new houses we built could have broken up any marriage, but we did it all for the girls and we survived.

The girls are older and more independent now. It's nice that Lauri and I have more time together. We enjoy going to movies, wine tasting, listening to bands, going for walks, shopping together, and having weekend getaways. Now that the girls are adults, some of these activities are even more fun when they join us. I'm really happy that Lindsey lives with us, but is also able to be independent. She and I enjoy the same type of TV comedy, but Lauri doesn't always agree with us. Lindsey is a big help around the house and makes great meals. We know this won't last. She wants to have her own apartment someday.

I still can't believe that I got Brittany to go bear hunting with me, and now we are even having a great time deer hunting together. We never thought we would see the day when the girls would become some of our best friends.

We both understand that we will never be free from autism or epilepsy. Recently Brittany had seizure activity at work, and we were able to have Lindsey pick her up and drive her to her house. Things like this remind us how far Lindsey has come. We will always work together, hopefully for many more years. We will never walk away.

Chapter Forty-Nine

"My Hopes and Dreams"

By Lindsey Moreland

"I figure life's a gift, and I don't intend on wasting it." - *Titanic, 1997*

"Life is like a box of chocolates, you never know what you're gonna get" -Forrest Gump, 1994

With this final chapter, readers will understand why I relate to those favorites quotes and how they explain my life. The first quote states how I really enjoy my life. I am glad to be the person that I am today. I didn't choose to be autistic. I was born this way. I am also grateful for my passions, but life isn't always that easy. When my parents and my sister share their memories of the negative stories of my autism, I sometimes feel sad. I sometimes feel offended and insulted if a person jokes about my autism. After learning about autism and how I behaved in the past, I wish I could change the past, but I can't do that because I can only change the future. I have been reassured lots of times by my family that it wasn't my fault on how I acted and I couldn't help it. I feel better when they mention that to me.

I want to continue being a motivational speaker, like Temple Grandin, by traveling across the United States and sharing what it is like having autism. I want to help other families with their struggles of autism. I still want to be an advocate against bullying. I was grateful that I started the SOS Program (Students Offering Support) at my high school to help other students not be excluded like I was. I want to help other school districts make a difference. I even want to be a guest speaker to teach children about autism, so they will become better educated about it. I want people to learn how to accept and appreciate others, positively. The quote that people of all ages should hear is **"Be Kind to One Another,"** by Ellen DeGeneres.

I have so many dreams that I hope to accomplish someday. First, I am adventurous. I would love to travel to places of my interests. I want to tour places where I have never been. Here are the top five destinations that are part of my bucket list: Spain, London, Paris, Italy, and New York City. So far, I have traveled to Florida twice, California, Mexico, and Canada. I went on a backpacking trip to the Superior Hiking Trail in 2015. That was quite an experience, lifting a 40 pound backpack while hiking, and going up and down the steep hills! But it was all worth it!

Second, I am a hard worker. I hope to find a paraprofessional job near my home, and find the school district that suits me well. However, if there are no openings yet, I can always find a different career. If it's meant to be, it's meant to be.

Third, the second quote states that life if full of surprises. In November 2016, I was officially in a relationship with my boyfriend. This is truly unexpected because I thought I wouldn't be in a relationship due to my autism. My boyfriend also has autism. That makes our relationship even more special because we understand each other and we have a lot in common. He hardly talks about his autism and I can respect that. As sensitive as we are, we hold hands, hug each other, and sometimes give each other kisses. We both love watching movies, drawing, going out for walks, and much more. I am thankful that his family has supported him gratefully as much as my family has for me. He is kind, mature, respectful, and has a great personality. I have my own box of pictures of us, and the cards he has given me from special holidays and other special occasions. I even have my own journal about our relationship and keep track of our dates. Every time I'm with him, he always puts a smile on my face and makes my day even happier.

Depending where I am with my relationship, I have a dream to marry someone special and live independently. With my independence, I continue being a pencil artist and enjoy my hobbies. I will also continue to eat healthy and exercise normally. I do not think I want to have children because having kids is expensive and overwhelming. I also don't want to go through a painful pregnancy and labor. However, with a paraprofessional job and my volunteering experiences, I do love working with children. I may find a different job, though.

Finally, I have a dream to meet Ellen DeGeneres someday. She inspires me and has taught us how to be kind, caring, and appreciative to others. She teaches how to be selfless, not selfish. She gives people the chance to share their amazing, inspiring stories, and talents. She helps people around the world with their struggles. She even has interviews with celebrities and their lifestyles. I enjoy laughing with her jokes and her good sense of humor! I sometimes feel like Ellen and I have the same personality because of how I care about other people, how I speak and teach people about autism, and how I made a difference at my school district.

In conclusion, I am truly grateful that I have a caring and fun-loving family who supports me. I am grateful to have Brittany as not only my sister, but my best friend. I am definitely thankful for my boyfriend and his family. I am happy to have a great personality, and be a person who is considered hard working, selfless, respectful, responsible, kind, caring, mature, quirky, funny, and appreciative. I continue to share my passions with other people. Without my family and friends, I wouldn't be the person I am today.

Chapter 50

"I'm not done yet."

By Lauri Moreland, Lindsey's mom

It was early August, my sister Linda had already been working hard in her classroom, preparing for the upcoming school year and her new students. We had set a goal for this book to be completed by the time she started back to work. I wanted our book to have a fairy tale ending. I wanted to be able to write that Lindsey had a full time job in the education field. Life doesn't always give you what you expect or want. After several years of very hard work and achieving her goals, Lindsey had built an impressive resume. She had applied for 6 jobs, received 5 interviews, and 5 rejections. As a mom, I saw all of her strengths and not her weaknesses. I thought she had proved her abilities when she volunteered 40 hours per week for an entire school year. Her volunteer work was spread out amongst three different elementary schools in three different districts.

I found out over the summer that some of the teachers that she had volunteered for had expressed concerns with Lindsey's ability to understand and follow through with directions. Unfortunately, they didn't always have the time to restate the directions or clarify the expectations for Lindsey. In addition, I did not find out about their concerns until the summer. I was feeling defeated, tired, and most of all sorry for Lindsey.

Yes, many people have to receive a lot of rejections before they finally get a "yes". It definitely made me realize that I am not done yet. I thought Lindsey would be able to get a job all on her own, and that I would not have to help her. Lindsey has more gifts and talents than I do. She wants so badly to have a paying job like the rest of us. She wants to buy her own car, rent her own apartment, and buy her groceries. She wants to travel the world. Plain and simple, Lindsey wants to be independent. This is what Todd and I have always wanted for both of our girls.

Sadly, not every parent will realize the dream of independence for their child. Although, when possible, I would hope that all children would be given the chance to work towards independence in adulthood.

I thought about it day and night. How were we going to get her employed? Previously stated, we sought guidance and help from the government program titled DVR which helps people with disabilities get employed. Lindsey and I had attended a meeting at the local library along with eight other people needing employment. Some of them were there with family members while others were there with their caretaker. We were all told about the program and that the process can take up to three months to be approved. It was so hard to wait and difficult to watch Lindsey's self-esteem deteriorate daily. In her words, "Without a job, I feel like a nobody."

The interviews Lindsey went on were about 20 minutes long. A short interview clearly does not demonstrate everything she is capable of doing. I know this because I went on an interview with her as a last resort. I called the local Y.M.C.A. after hearing that they are an accepting place of employment for adults with special needs. I pleaded my case with them. They kindly set up an interview for Lindsey in which I could attend. They wanted to meet both of us.

As I sat and listened in on the interview, I was completely shocked. Some of the questions she was asked were not anything she was prepared for. Some of her answers did not make sense at all. My brain wandered as I now understood what the teachers were talking about. It was difficult for me not to step in and correct her answers.

In our everyday lives, I still have to explain some things to Lindsey an extra time or two. I am completely ok with it and used to it. So, this shouldn't have been a shock to me. I never thought about how this would affect her ability to work or get her employed. Now I wondered, "Who would take the extra time or have the patience needed when Lindsey didn't understand a direction or task? Who would give her a chance to prove that she would be a great employee?"

We live in a fast, ever changing world. I look around and notice how little time and patience people have for one another. The news and various studies show how stressed out, tired, and overwhelmed we are as a society. It is easy to forget that many people, not just those diagnosed with autism, could benefit from repeated directions and a "show not tell" approach. I find myself guilty of this as well. It is easier for me to give a haircut than take the time to explain what I am doing or show how I am doing it. However, this is what Lindsey needs. She needs an employer who is willing to slow down and take the time to coach and teach her at her level of processing. We left the interview, and we were both excited. I felt like the Y.M.C.A would be the perfect employer for Lindsey. I felt like she could be successful working for them.

The manager told us that we would find out by the end of the week. The wait was longer than expected and turned into almost three weeks. During this time, we started to lose hope. I began talking to people about my concerns with getting not only Lindsey employed, but also other adults on the spectrum. With one in sixty-eight people now living on the autism spectrum, our society will need to figure out how to help these individuals be successful in the workplace. Not all, but many of these individuals are capable of working.

In my frustration, I wanted to hop in the car, drive to Madison, and knock on every government employee door I could find. Congressmen, senators, or the governor himself...I wanted my concerns heard. This is a major crisis for parents who have adults with autism. Within our circle of friends, I know of adults with autism or other special needs who are living in their parents' basement, defeated, depressed, and on the verge of giving up. It breaks my heart when I know they just need and deserve a chance. Collecting disability from the government is not the chance they are looking for in their lives. They want a real job. A common challenge for people with autism is the social part of our world. This carries over as a challenge in the workplace. In Lindsey's case, she can give a clear, confident, excellent speech to hundreds of people without any problem while maintaining eye contact. However, a job in which she would have to interact with hundreds of people throughout the day would give her anxiety and excessive stress, leading to physical ailments.

As the days went by and we still heard nothing from the Y.M.C.A., I cried a lot. I talked to my mom, my sister, and my friends. I boldly stated, "I am losing hope again!" It seems like when I am just about ready to throw in the towel, something happens that helps the situation get a little better. We received a letter in the mail from DVR, the government program, stating that Lindsey had been approved to receive help in getting a job. Three days later, before DVR got involved, we received a call from the Y.M.C.A. They wanted more information about Lindsey. I was able to talk to the manager, and she said Lindsey could expect a call within a few days.

As I write this, today is September 15, 2017. Today is the day Lindsey got that sweet call telling her to bring her driver's license, her social security number, and birth certificate to the Y.M.C.A. on this upcoming Monday. They are giving her a job. If she needs a job coach, she will get one from the government program.

I have my fairy tale ending, for now. She is joyful, motivated, and happy to start this next chapter in her life. Our story continues with many unknowns, numerous goals accomplished, and a positive outlook for the future.

Epilogue

"Final Thoughts"

By Lauri Moreland, Lindsey's mom

As a mom who gave birth to a child with autism, I want to share some insight and advice for other parents who have felt criticized or judged for their parenting decisions. Throughout the years, I have heard it all. Your child's okay because:

"My kid has tantrums!"

"My kid doesn't eat well either."

"My kid didn't start talking until later."

"My child doesn't sleep well."

"My kid spins."

"My child is a toe walker.

"Do you think he has autism?"

"My kid is obsessed with movies, too."

"Just take the movies away.

"It's not good to let your child watch so much TV."

"Your child still has a pacifier?"

"Your 4 year old isn't potty trained yet?"

"You can't give her everything she wants."

"You can't change her schedule? Really?"

"Maybe she just needs a good

 - old fashioned spanking."

"She looks so normal."

"Just give her a time out!"

"I am sure that she will grow out of this."

"My child cries a lot,

 (probably) just as much as yours."

"My kid doesn't like haircuts either."

"My child throws toys, too."

"Are you sure she is autistic?"

"Is she still autistic?"

The list could go on and on. Then, there were all the stares and the dirty looks when we were in public. There was eye rolling, annoyed body language, faces, and sighs. I developed a very tough skin. At times, I wished Lindsey had a shirt that said, "I have autism-don't look at me."

My advice to others is to trust yourself and trust that feeling that something is not right with your child regardless of what others say, believe, or do. Seek out the help immediately. Don't second guess yourself because in my opinion early intervention is essential. Get second opinions and third opinions if you think you need them. Lean on family and friends who support you in a positive way. Do your best to avoid negative opinions because it feels toxic. Figure out ways to take time for yourself and don't blame yourself or let others blame you. Hopefully at some point you can find humor in the unique ways your child sees the world. Admit that you can't do it all or do it alone, and never give up. For us, I believe that the best is yet to come.

The process of writing this book has been extremely emotional for our family. There have been many tears, but many laughs, too. It has been a healing journey for Todd, Brittany, Lindsey, and me. Hours and hours have been spent watching home videos along with reading medical and educational paperwork. I am grateful that I saved it all. We've spent many hours and days being interviewed by our co-author, my sister, Linda Wagner.

The process has been different for all of us. Lindsey would write her chapters in her own private space. She would meet with Linda at coffee shops or our house to edit. Brittany would sit side by side with Linda on the majority of her chapters. Sometimes, after reading a chapter, she would go home and add more. Todd was always interviewed by Linda in our kitchen. It was the first time I ever saw him have an emotional reaction to our past years dealing with Lindsey's autism. In fact, there are many things that we never discussed until this book. My mom, Grandma Ida, wrote her chapters at home and then submitted them to Linda. For me, this over two year endeavor has often been all consuming. I have lost sleep and so has Linda due to the stress and honesty of it all.

Linda and I have probably spent the most time together in all of our childhood and adult years. We have worked on chapters during walks, at coffee shops, at our house, and over the phone. We have had challenging conversations over feelings, experiences, and memories. It is not easy to dig up the past, especially when it hurts. Yet, we have all done our best to present ourselves in the most honest way possible realizing that it may not please or be easy to read for some of our family and friends.

In this published version, we have changed a few names and taken out names of school districts and towns. As times change and the years go by, there is more and more information about autism. I hold no anger towards any school district and completely understand that educating students with autism years ago was a lot different than it is today.

As I look ahead to how I can advocate for not only Lindsey, but also other adults with special needs, I beg you to join me on a mission to figure out a way to provide these adults with employment opportunities. People from all walks of life are living this. We need to go out and talk to employers. We need to get employers educated and help them see the benefits of hiring our children who are now adults. Keep pushing for this kind of diversity in the workplace. Talk to your congressmen and other government representatives in your community.

I am grateful for all of the people in our lives that have supported us in every way including family, friends, educators, therapists, and strangers who smiled and offered help. I will never forget the day I was at a store with Lindsey when something suddenly set her off into a screaming tantrum in the checkout line. Struggling to carry the bags and Lindsey out to the car, a sweet woman approached me and offered to help me. Her eyes were kind and her smile was gentle. She did not judge me, and she wasn't annoyed. I never got her name, nor did I probably thank her enough. She was my angel at the time. My hope is that as you read these final words, **you** will be that family member, that friend, that educator, that therapist, or that stranger that is making a positive difference in the life of a child and a family.

LIVE – SURVIVE – THRIVE

By sharing our family story of living with autism and mental health concerns, we hope to inspire others to live, survive, and thrive in today's society. Our mission is to share our story through our book, speaking engagements, and consulting with families.

We encourage you to follow the Moreland family story on our website. Check out information on upcoming events, see Lindsey's artwork, and pictures of our family. Email us if you are interested in ordering books, t-shirts designed by Lindsey, or talking to us about booking a speaking engagement.

Website: autismlm.com
Email: autismlm@gmail.com